Cleanse
Your System

D1081039

Cleanse
Your System

Find inner health through a unique
purification programme

Amanda Ursell

Thorsons
An Imprint of HarperCollins*Publishers*

While the author of this work has made every effort to ensure that the information contained in this book is as accurate and up to date as possible at the time of publication, medical knowledge is constantly changing and the application of it to particular circumstances depends on many factors. Therefore it is recommended that readers always consult a qualified medical specialist for individual advice. This book should not be used as an alternative to seeking specialist medical advice, which should be sought before any action is taken. The author and publishers cannot be held responsible for any errors and omissions that may be found in the text, or any actions that may be taken by a reader as a result of any reliance on the information contained in the text, which is taken entirely at the reader's own risk.

The author would like to thank Warner Wellcome for the use of data from their NOP survey on indigestion, in Chapter 9.

Thorsons
An Imprint of HarperCollins*Publishers*
77–85 Fulham Palace Road,
Hammersmith, London W6 8JB

Published by Thorsons 1999

3 5 7 9 10 8 6 4 2

© Amanda Ursell 1999

Amanda Ursell asserts the moral right to
be identified as the author of this work

Text illustrations by Peter Cox

A catalogue record for this book
is available from the British Library

ISBN 0 7225 3843 X

Printed and bound in Great Britain by
Caledonian International Book Manufacturing Ltd, Glasgow

For my parents and for Stuart

Contents

— 1 —

The Digestive System

Perhaps the best way to start this book is by telling you what it is *not* about. First, it is not about to start recommending you organize 10 colonic irrigation sessions to manually wash out your insides. Nor will it demand that you to start following some mad detoxification plan which leaves you starving in the mistaken belief that such emptiness must by implication be cleaning you out. Instead, *Cleanse Your System* is about understanding the reality of what goes on in your digestive system on a daily basis. By looking at what and when we eat, and how our emotional and psychological well-being play very direct roles in our digestive health, we learn to discover how to cleanse and calm our digestive systems – naturally.

The Sensitive Gut

Physically, your digestive tract is really just one long tube which is surrounded by muscles. This tube takes on different shapes and roles as it makes its way through the body from the mouth down into the throat, the stomach, on into the small and large intestine and finally to the rectum and anus.

This muscular tube cannot function on its own. To be able to break large pieces of food into smaller ones, mix them with various enzymes and acids, kill off the harmful bacteria and bugs we eat in our food, dispose of waste material and, finally, allow the absorption of useful nutrients into the bloodstream ... there needs to be a very efficient Commanding Officer.

The digestive system's CO comes in the form of its very own nervous system, known as the Enteric Nervous System or ENS. The ENS communicates with the rest of the body and our brains via a huge and complex set of nerves (almost as many as in the brain itself). This means that what is going on in the gut affects our brain, and equally, what is going on in our brain affects our gut.

In practice this means the gut can tell the brain what to do and how to behave, and the brain can have direct effects on telling the gut what to do. Take the fact that simply looking at and smelling an appetizing meal can stimulate the flow of saliva. What has happened to elicit this response is that your senses of sight and smell have stimulated the brain. The brain has then sent a message to the ENS to tell it food is on its way and to start producing saliva in the mouth and acid in the stomach to get in preparation for the food which it believes is about to arrive.

Then there is the situation where the gut's nervous system tells the ENS something and the brain responds. For example, once some food such as meat enters the small intestine, the ENS sends a message to the brain telling it that some protein-breaking enzymes need to be released. The brain sends a message back to the gut which stimulates the release of some of the appropriate enzymes.

Emotional Responses

When we get upset about something or worried about a particular situation, such as taking a driving test, speaking in front of a roomful of people or starting a new job, the brain can play havoc with the ENS, sending messages which make the entire tract start contracting – leading, for example, to 'butterflies in the stomach', a nauseous feeling or even a heavy bout of loose stools.

Digestion – What the Process Involves

Year in, year out, adults munch their way through a good 500 kg (about 1 lb) of food each day. That's equivalent to the weight of seven men! Never before in history have we consumed such a huge array of different foods and drinks, and never before have we done so at such an extraordinary pace of life.

Each day we ask our digestive systems to deal with the processing of a huge variety of chemical substances, from the useful nutrients in foods and drinks to unfriendly bacteria and viruses and non-nutrient material which must be expelled from the system. Each section of the system has very distinct functions, and in turn suffers very distinct problems when things get out of kilter.

For much of the time we are blissfully unaware that our digestive systems are just getting on with the daily grind of transforming everything that enters our mouths into useful small-sized nutrients which can be absorbed, rendering harmful substances safe or separating out what is not needed and disposing of it as waste, either in our urine or stools.

These extraordinarily complex processes are, as already described, under the influence of the ENS and brain, along with quite a few chemical messengers known as hormones.

These processes are taking place all the time. We expect our digestive systems to keep on processing everything we throw at them without complaint.

That sometimes things go wrong – perhaps we suffer with a bout of heartburn, some trapped wind or something more problematic and long-term like Irritable Bowel Syndrome – is not surprising. There comes a point when the mix, quantities and pace at which we eat and drink can send our digestive systems into turmoil. At this point they start to rebel, letting us know in no uncertain terms that it is time for a break, time to think about

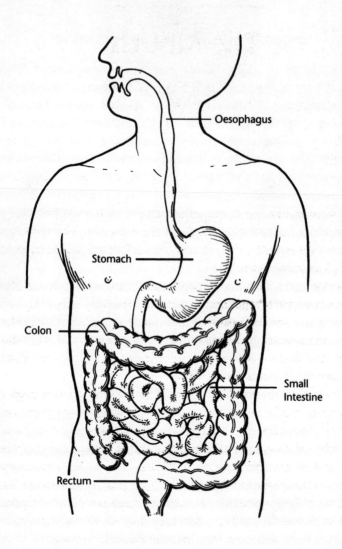

Figure 1 The digestive tract

restoring some balance and helping ourselves to a calmer, more peaceful internal existence.

2

The Mouth

Undoubtedly the most enjoyable part of eating and drinking occurs in the mouth, where food and drink first enter the body. It's here that we experience the textures and flavours that register as being pleasurable in the brain.

Just the sight and smell of food stimulate the brain to tell the nerves of the gut to begin producing saliva from the many salivary glands which line the inside of the mouth and cheeks. Once the flow has started and you actually get a delicious morsel into your mouth, the sheer mechanical action of physically chewing food stimulates further saliva production.

This is where the need for a good clean digestive system begins and where, if it is not achieved and maintained, poor digestion starts. A copious flow of saliva is crucial not only to the chewing and swallowing of food, but also to the cleanliness and condition of the teeth and gums. Tooth decay and gum disease are surprisingly common reasons for indigestion, and a lack of saliva increases the risk of both. Poor standards of oral cleanliness can also be responsible for bad breath, which immediately gives others the impression your digestive system could benefit from a quick spring-clean.

Saliva Production

In one day alone it is quite normal to produce over a litre (more than 1 gallon) of saliva. At rest we make about 0.5 ml (about ¼oz) per minute, which increases significantly on eating. Sucking a lemon (just the thought makes your mouth water), can cause a 100-fold rise in saliva flow.

A good flow of saliva physically helps clean the teeth and gums of chewed food by washing them away. The enzyme lysozyme, contained in saliva, helps to destroy potentially harmful bacteria, while the mucus coats chewed food so that when it moves on to be swallowed the oesophagus is protected from being scratched and damaged. Saliva also helps you to distinguish and enjoy flavours by dissolving components of foods which stimulate the taste buds.

A reduction in saliva production may be due to dehydration. Once you become thirsty it a sure sign that your body is already dehydrated and needs topping up with fluids as quickly as possible. This is a good survival mechanism because a dry mouth due to reduced saliva production brought on by dehydration is the strongest stimulus we have for searching out fluids to redress the imbalance.

Saliva flow is also severely restricted at times of severe mental effort and fear. Being uptight and worried when you eat can become a vicious circle, since a poor saliva flow makes eating less enjoyable, comfortable and tasty, which in turn can add to the stress of the experience.

That fear reduces salivary flow is well documented and has even been used as a crude test of a person's guilt or innocence in the 'Indian Rice Test'. A person unable to swallow dried rice was thought to be guilty on the grounds that fear prevents secretions. Goodness how many innocent people have been condemned on this basis. The fear of failing was probably enough to dry up any secretions they may have had.

Saliva and Tooth Decay

'Oh, I wish I'd looked after me teeth, and spotted the perils beneath,
all the toffees I'd chewed and the sweet sticky food, Oh, I wish I'd
looked after me teeth.'

So wrote Pam Ayres – a sentiment many of us echo as we endure the screeching of the dentist's drill. Keeping our teeth in good condition doesn't just save us from the horrors of the dental surgery, but aides digestion and promotes oral cleanliness.

Decay of the tooth occurs when remains of food eaten stick to the teeth and start forming plaque, a sticky substance which is an ideal breeding ground for the multiplication of bacteria which live in the mouth. The sugary substances in plaque are fermented by these bacteria, which produce acid – it is this acid which causes the enamel of the tooth to break down, causing decay right through into the softer dentine layers below. If the next layer of the tooth, the pulp, is also attacked, abscesses can form.

We have known for some time that the key to preventing tooth decay is avoiding sugary snacks between meals and brushing teeth regularly after eating to remove the vestiges of food which lead to plaque. Producing adequate saliva is also vital.

Saliva is naturally alkali and provides the safest environment in which the teeth can be bathed. Stimulating salivary flow after a meal helps to wash away bits of food and returns the mouth to its preferred alkali state. Chewing gum after a meal is a good way of increasing salivary flow, restoring a high pH and reducing the risk of decay.

The most effective chewing gums are those containing the natural sweetener xylitol. Made from the birch tree, xylitol has been shown in clinical research to reduce the risk of tooth decay through a variety of mechanisms.

First, the xylitol increases salivary flow above and beyond the capacity of normal gums, thus helping to raise pH and neutralize acids even more rapidly. Secondly, it inhibits the growth of the bacteria (*streptococcus mutans*) which grow on plaque. It is the only natural sweetener that has this property. Thirdly, it helps reduce decay by reducing the quantity of plaque produced in the mouth, making it less adhesive to teeth and thus easier to clean off. Finally, xylitol helps to remineralize areas of enamel which have already been attacked. Not only this, it keeps your breath fresh. Xylitol is added to Wrigley's Extra chewing gum, blue Smints and a variety of mouthwashes and toothpastes such as Boots Total Care toothpaste.

Periodontal Disease

Periodontal (which means located around a tooth) disease starts, often during childhood, as inflammation of the gum margin, with redness, swelling and bleeding on brushing. It occurs as sticky deposits of plaque gather around the gum. As the gum swells through inflammation it causes a little trap for more plaque to grow in. At this stage the problem is known as gingivitis and can be reversed by effective oral hygiene. Without adequate dental hygiene, a second stage, chronic periodontitis, may develop in which the bone and fibres which support the teeth are progressively destroyed, leading to loosening and, finally, loss of the tooth.

The key to preventing and dealing with early stages of periodontal disease and tooth decay is to reduce plaque. Improving saliva flow to help remove plaque-forming material and restore a plaque-unfriendly environment is important. Again, chewing the right kind of gum can help.

Good personal care of the teeth prevents and helps treat this problem, which obviously has implications on the digestive process if left to progress. The gentle scrub technique used in brushing teeth with a fluoride toothpaste, flossing, disclosing plaque with tablets and the use of xylitol gum between meals can all help.

Other Roles of Saliva

In addition to the roles mentioned above, saliva also actually starts the breaking down of some nutrients. The enzyme amylase which is present in saliva begins the process of breaking down carbohydrates. Try chewing a piece of bread for a few minutes. As the salivary amylase enzymes start to work on the starch in the bread, they begin to turn into simple sugars which taste sweeter. The enzymes get to work on the surface of foods they come into contact with – so grinding food into very small particles in the mouth by chewing them thoroughly can promote this first stage of digestion. There is also a small amount of the enzyme which breaks down fat present in saliva.

Saliva is vital, too, for keeping the mouth moist to allow speech and oral comfort. A reduction in saliva production clearly has far-reaching consequences not just on the digestive processes and cleanliness of the mouth, but also on our ability to communicate easily and effectively.

Taking time to eat your food in peace and quiet, or at least giving yourself enough time to stop dashing and sit peacefully for a few minutes before you start, may help improve saliva flow if you are constantly on the go. Chewing slowly and thoroughly can help, as may mastering yoga breathing techniques. Trying to tempt people to eat who are down and have lost their appetite is not easy, but one way which may help is to stimulate saliva flow through good tastes and smells, hot, well-flavoured soups, an alcoholic apéritif or a mineral water with a splash of lime juice and a squeeze of lemon.

Halitosis

Typically caused by poor dental hygiene, and particularly by gingivitis, bad breath is a sure sign that your digestive system needs a spring clean. Try following the advice above. It is also worth making sure that your diet is rich in vitamin C – found in berries, citrus fruits, green peppers and dark green vegetables – plus beta carotene, found in carrots and dark red and green fruits and vegetables, to ensure any damaged and bleeding gums have the right nutrients to help rapid repair.

Also bear in mind that halitosis may also be due to disorders further down the digestive system, such as constipation and a change in gut bacterial flora. It is possible that the use of probiotics which restore good bacteria to the large intestine may help (see Chapter 6).

3

The Oesophagus

Once food has been chewed and mixed with saliva, it's time to swallow the masticated lumps into the first real 'tubular' part of the digestive tract, known as the oesophagus.

Swallowing is where the tongue springs into action. We swallow literally hundreds of times a day without giving a thought to just how complicated a process it is. In the way we learned during weaning, the tongue rises up and presses against the roof of the mouth. This forces the lump of food – or bolus as it's called in technical terms – into the back of the throat. This series of movements alone involves around 22 separate muscle groups. From here, rather like when you go to a fun fair and sit on the big dipper, once the starter switch has been pressed there's no going back.

The bolus is swept into the back of the throat (called the pharynx), an action that triggers nerves to tell the muscles surrounding the oesophagus to contract and relax in wavelike patterns. These pulsating movements carry the bolus like a raft on the rapids, downwards to the stomach.

The entire journey from mouth to stomach is remarkably quick, taking just four to eight seconds. Fluids travel even faster, whizzing through this part of the journey in one to two seconds.

To stop the bolus taking a wrong turning and shooting off into the windpipe instead of making its way on into the stomach, a small flap closes over the entrance to the windpipe to block it off.

If you try to talk or inhale while swallowing, the protective mechanisms can be disrupted and short-circuited, with food getting into the breathing passageways. If this happens, frantic coughing is triggered, which is the body's way of trying to expel the food as quickly as possible and stop you choking.

Throughout its meandering course through the body, the digestive system is punctuated by valves and 'gateways'. The first of these is situated just above the entrance to the stomach. Known as the lower oesophageal valve, it too is closed off until it detects the approach of the bolus making its way down the oesophagus. As the bolus gets close to the top of the stomach, the muscular valve, acting as a gateway, opens, allowing the lump of food to continue on into the stomach, the bag-like storage tank of the digestive system.

The stomach environment is highly acidic and its lining is specially adapted to cope with the very corrosive nature of its contents. Other parts of the digestive tract lining the oesophagus are not acidic. It is quite normal for the valve which separates the oesophagus from the stomach to allow small amounts of the acidy contents to leak back up, they are then simply washed back into the stomach by regular swallowing of saliva. Some people suffer with severe reflux of their acidic stomach contents, which actually burns the oesophagus lining leading to the age-old cause of indigestion – heartburn. This is dealt with in more detail in Chapter 4.

Oesophageal Irritability

Another sensation which manifests itself as a pain in the chest, but is neither caused by heartburn nor serious heart problems, is oesophageal irritability, which may simply be caused by the muscular waves of the oesophagus getting out of kilter. Drinking very cold, very hot or carbonated drinks can all evoke odd and uncomfortable contractions. Even a loud noise like the sudden clapping of the hands can create this response in the oesophagus.

It has also been long suspected that an irritable oesophagus is related to emotional stress, anxiety or depression. Even setting someone tricky tasks in the school or work environment can be held responsible for sending the throat into uncomfortable spasm. Treating the root of the emotional stress may well help to relieve the physical indigestion it causes.

A Lump in the Throat

As well as an irritable oesophagus upsetting digestion, the feeling that you have a lump in your throat may have similar effects. It often comes between, rather that at, mealtimes, and tends to occur just below the Adam's apple level. It is noticeable during periods of strong emotions, often disappearing when you cry, but if left untreated can affect smooth swallowing and reduce the desire to eat.

It has been suggested that these lumps in the throat occur more often in tense people who swallow repeatedly, which creates a dry mouth and then the lump. Becoming 'choked up' with grief, disappointment or pride can also contract the throat muscles in an uncoordinated fashion, leading to further discomfort. Interestingly, a lump in the throat is often relieved by eating, drinking, having a good cry or seeking help to calm your under-lying emotional tensions and worries.

Other Problems

A goitre occurs when the thyroid gland (situated in the throat) swells, leading to difficulties with swallowing as the goitre presses on the oesophagus, restricting its width. This is a problem that your doctor will need to treat.

The wide range of potential causes of digestive problems associated with the throat means that it is vital that any difficulties with swallowing be checked out by your doctor.

Action Plan

Dietary Advice

Once your doctor has identified the problem, advice on what to eat to keep nutrient intakes up is important. If swallowing needs to be relearned, then the help of both a speech therapist and a dietitian is invaluable.

Generally, the best foods to try if swallowing is a problem are those that are soft, need little chewing and will slip down easily. Chilled soft foods, like ice-cream, jellies, smooth yogurt, fromage frais, mousses and thick custards are good starting points. Slightly chilled foods are good, too, because they stimulate the swallowing reflex more easily than do warm ones. This is because there are more receptors that register cold temperatures at the back of the mouth than there are that register warm ones.

As swallowing improves, then you can move on to mixed-consistency foods.

Emotional Stress

Dealing with emotional stress is very important. See advice in Chapter 8.

Herbal Remedies

See Chapter 8.

4

The Stomach

The stomach is the point at which the digestive tract forms itself into a pouch and acts as a temporary reservoir. While it is possible to survive without a stomach, it does carry out some important digestive processes.

During the course of your life, your stomach learns to accept a bewildering array of lumps of food and a wide variety of drinks. A bolus (lump of food) may be hard, soft, acidic, alkaline, watery or solid. Whatever form each bolus takes when it enters the stomach, by the time it's ready to go on into the small intestine it needs to have been turned from a solid into a liquid, and that liquid needs to be of a consistent pH – in other words, not too acidic and not too alkaline. To ensure this, the stomach carries out several functions.

Like the rest of the digestive tract, the stomach is surrounded by lots of muscles. It can vary in shape a little from one person to another, but is generally a 'J'-shaped bag (see Figure 2). In short, stout people it tends to run horizontally, whereas in tall, thin people the J is more vertical.

In either type of person, the stomach is surprisingly high up and not by the belly button, which is normally where we point to if complaining of stomach ache. When we are not eating (for example at night and for about four hours after the last meal), the stomach is relatively empty and looks like a deflated balloon, about 25 cm (10 in) long. In this state, it holds about 50 ml

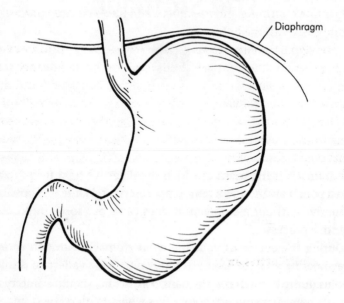

Diaphragm

Figure 2 Diagram of the stomach, shaped like a 'J'-shaped bag

(2 fl oz), one third of a small yogurt pot. Once full, however, it can really expand, holding up to 4 litres (7 pints) of food and drink. This comes in handy for feast days, highdays and holidays when we usually overindulge. After a normal meal, it would contain more like 1.5 to 2 litres (2½ to 3½ pints).

One of the stomach's main roles is to put the muscles surrounding it into action. By contracting and relaxing, they set up a powerful churning motion, like a cement mixer, grinding and mixing its contents. Just as a builder would add water to thin a cement mix down, so the body secretes mucus and gastric juices, produced in copious quantities in the stomach wall. Nerves and hormones take the role of the builder controlling these additions, but these in turn are under the control of the foreman, the brain, which judges carefully how much of each needs to be added. The churning continues and the mucus and juices become thoroughly combined with the bolus.

The signal to start secreting, as we have seen, is given as soon as we see, smell or even think about food – a sort of advance party, letting the stomach know it's on standby. Once food and drink actually hit the stomach, more juices pour in from the walls of the stomach – partly in response to its physical presence, and partly due to the chemical make-up of the bolus it receives. The mucus that pours in is alkaline. It coats the stomach wall as well as mixing with the food and softening it up.

The juices contain three substances:

1. hydrochloric acid, which lowers the pH of the stomach environment and kills bugs
2. pepsin, which is an enzyme that helps digest protein
3. hormones, which control the contractions and movement of the muscular stomach.

The hydrochloric acid is extremely strong. When secreted, it immediately makes the stomach contents very acidic, with a pH of between 1.5 and 3.5 (neutral is pH 7). These acidic conditions are needed to help in the digestion of proteins and to kill off the many bacteria that enter the stomach in and with food and drink. Due to its low pH, hydrochloric acid is highly corrosive, apparently more so than the acid in a car battery, so that if the contents of the stomach were placed on a wooden table, they would bore their way through.

The acid clearly has a vital role, but the stomach wall has to be protected from it to avoid being damaged itself. Like most parts of the body when they are functioning properly, it has developed ways of getting round the potential problem. It does so in several ways. First, it has a thick coating of the alkaline mucus built up over it. Second, the cells of the stomach lining are very tightly cemented together, preventing gastric juices leaking into the tissues below. Third, if cells are damaged, they are quickly shed and replaced. The lining is completely shed and renewed every three to six days anyway to ensure that only fresh protective cells are in place.

The nerves and hormones that control the secretions and movements communicate directly with the brain. The brain controls the movements and secretions by detecting the physical presence and chemical compostion of food in the stomach via the nerves and hormones. The brain also affects the stomach's movements in response to external stimuli. Any form of anxiety, stress, emotional turmoil, fright or depression will be detected in the brain and exert their effect, through the nerves, on the stomach. In times of intense stress, for example, it's unlikely that you will feel the need to eat and so you can lose your appetite. The link between how we feel and the effect this has on all parts of the digestive tract should never be underestimated.

Certain components and nutrients in food and drink that enter the stomach can also directly affect the secretion of mucus and juice, and the valves at the top and bottom of the stomach.

Alcohol, aspirin and water are virtually the only substances that are absorbed directly from the stomach into the bloodstream – the rest must pass on into the small intestine.

Over a period of a few hours, the bolus will have gradually been broken down into a liquidy substance known as chyme. This has to pass out of the stomach and on into the first section of the small intestine, called the duodenum.

Problems with the Stomach

Heartburn

Heartburn is one of the commonest forms of indigestion, and the one people are usually describing when they complain of an 'acidy' taste in the throat and/or mouth. Heartburn occurs when the acid contents of the stomach spill back, past the sphincter into the gullet or oesophagus. On occasions, they may actually reflux right the way back and up into the mouth.

It's important to get the idea of reflux into perspective. Small amounts of reflux are actually perfectly normal and happen to most of us, most of the time. The muscular valve or gateway to the stomach allows some of the acidic mix of half-digested food to leak back out. It is in particularly susceptible people and those in whom large quantities seep out that the problem is both painful in the short term and a potential problem in the long term.

When you stop and think about it, it's hardly surprising that heartburn hurts. The stomach is equipped to deal with the acidic nature of its contents by having a thick, duvet-like coating of mucus to protect its surface. As we saw in Chapter 3, the oesophagus has no such protection. Swallowing saliva, which is alkaline, can help to neutralize the normal, small amounts of regurgitated acidic material, and the swallowing action itself helps to sweep these stomach contents back down to where they belong. If any is left, however, or reflux gets out of hand, the acid can literally start digesting the surface cells of the gullet and back of the throat. This is what causes the nerves to register pain.

Heartburn is most likely to occur when the valves at the top of the stomach and bottom of the gullet become weakened (see Figure 3). This is common in pregnancy when, it is believed, the extra levels of the hormone progesterone that are circulating have this weakening effect. Smoking is also thought to loosen the sphincter, as are certain drugs.

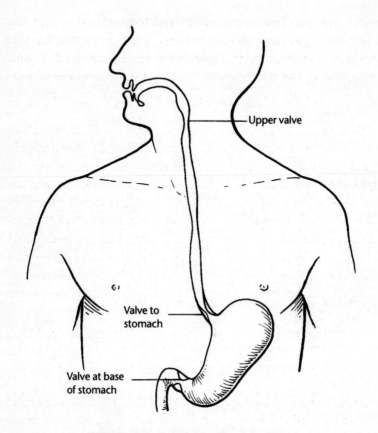

Figure 3 The valves of the gullet and stomach.

In other cases, the sphincter may be perfectly fit, but the pressure of, say, bending or lying down or lifting something heavy can overcome its ability to hold the stomach contents in and so leakage follows. Lying down soon after eating can lead to acid reflux, too. The stomach is physically tipped up and some of its contents forced past the valve and into the gullet.

Constipation, perhaps rather surprisingly, can cause reflux from the stomach into the gullet, too. When you strain to go to the toilet, the pressure builds up in the large intestine and has nowhere to go except back up the tract. The end result is that this pressure is relieved by the opening of the stomach valve, with reflux being the consequence. This is a good example of how something going wrong in one part of the gut can indirectly affect another part.

Extra pressure within the abdominal cavity has an adverse effect on sphincter strength as well. Pregnant women suffer not only from the effects of progesterone chemically weakening the sphincter, but from the foetus pushing the stomach and its contents up and, once again, forcing the stomach's contents up and out of the top of the intestinal sack. This is especially likely to occur during the last trimester and making changes to diet and lifestyle are the only steps that can be taken to help relieve this kind of heartburn (these are detailed below). The accumulation of fat in the abdominal cavity in both overweight and obese people has the same effect.

Certain foods can affect the strength of this gateway to the stomach. Fats, for example, seem to relax the muscle tone of the sphincter, as do coffee, alcohol, onions, garlic, peppermints and chocolates.

Very large meals – which not only fill the stomach to capacity, but also sit around for hours and take ages to digest – will often lead to reflux. This is usually an infrequent cause of problems, occurring at, say, Christmas, special parties and dinners and so on, and so shouldn't be unduly worried over. It is just nature's way of letting you know you've overdone it.

Heartburn is made worse in susceptible people by severe emotional upset. The brain-gut connection reacts, with fear, anxiety and anger stimulating reflux.

Above the stomach, there sits a big band of muscle separating the stomach from the lungs. Called the diaphragm, it is possible for the top part of the stomach to push up and through this muscular barrier, creating a hiatus hernia (see Figure 4). Quite a few sufferers experience reflux and heartburn as a result of having a hernia.

In a few people, the refluxing of the stomach's contents into the gullet can lead to inflammation. Severe cases may result in bleeding, which, if it carries on over a period of time, can lead to anaemia. The inflammation, or oesophagitis as it's known, may eventually cause scarring and a narrowing of the gullet. This is obviously uncomfortable and may ultimately lead to cancer.

As you can see, it is vital that any serious refluxing is reported to your doctor, who may decide to investigate and look into things further. An investigation with an endoscope might be

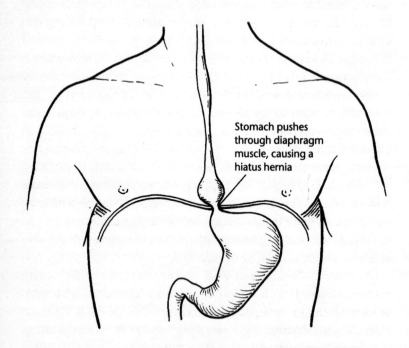

Stomach pushes through diaphragm muscle, causing a hiatus hernia

Figure 4 How a hiatus hernia is formed.

recommended, which involves swallowing a narrow tube – the endoscope – which has a camera and light in the end to enable the doctor to have a good look around and also take little tissue samples from the gullet to study under a microscope later.

There is a plethora of drugs and remedies available on prescription from the doctor or over the counter at the chemist's for heartburn. Equally, there are many positive dietary and lifestyle improvements you can make that can help to reduce the number and severity of attacks.

Dietary Advice

How and when you eat cannot be separated from the chemical composition of the food and drink itself in terms of the effects on your digestive system.

First of all, always try to make time to eat and drink and avoid, whenever possible, doing either when on the go. Sit down and leave yourself time, however short of it you are.

Chewing thoroughly is also important. It not only gets the digestive process off to a good start by thoroughly mixing in enzymes and turning food into small and easy-to-swallow pieces, it helps avoid the 'bolting' down of a meal or snack.

If you make yourself calm prior to eating and take the whole process at a more leisurely pace, your nervous system will calm down and produce less acid in the stomach.

Timings and Quantities

It's best to avoid huge influxes of food and drink at any one time to reduce the risk of overfilling the stomach. The stomach holds 1.5 litres (2½ pints) comfortably without becoming badly overextended. If too much is eaten at one go, the stomach becomes overfull, it cannot empty itself fast enough to clear it and reflux is likely.

This means it's important not to skip meals, only to overindulge several hours later. Small, regular intakes – such as a light breakfast, mid morning snack, lunch, mid-afternoon snack and finally a light evening meal – is the best pattern to adopt to avoid reflux and heartburn. It is vital that you leave time after your last meal of the day for the food to start moving from the stomach into the intestine – in other words, a good few hours before going to bed. The risk of *not* following such a rule is that, as soon as you lie down, the contents of the stomach move into the oesophagus by sheer virtue of gravity. So, why deliberately make things worse for yourself?

The Chemical Composition of Foods

Certain components of foods and drinks can actually weaken the sphincter at the top of the stomach.

Protein-rich meals seem to enhance the tone of the valve, making it tighter and, therefore, a better blocker. Good sources of protein include lean meat, poultry without the skin, fish (white and oily), eggs and reduced-fat dairy products, such as milk and cheese.

Fatty foods have quite the opposite effect. Meals and snacks rich in fat *relax* the sphincter, making reflux and therefore heartburn in susceptible people more likely. Most people in the West consume more calories than necessary from fats and would be well advised to reduce their totals for other health reasons. Diets rich in fat are more likely to lead to putting on weight. If high in saturated fatty acids, they can increase cholesterol levels in the blood and thus the risk of heart disease.

Fats have another action on the stomach that can make heartburn more likely. When a fat-rich bolus reaches the stomach, small bits of it are passed on into the top part of the small intestine. In this section, the duodenum, it is recognized that the fat content is high, which stimulates the release of a hormone called enterogastrin. This hormone acts as a messenger and tells the muscles of the stomach to slow down its contractions. With the movements of the muscles reduced, the mixing and grinding takes longer and food stays in the stomach for greater periods of time. In those who suffer refluxes, the time period over which it could occur is therefore increased as a fatty meal can remain in the stomach for up to four or five hours.

Cutting back on fat is important from a weight point of view, too. As mentioned, fatty diets tend to lead to weight gain. Gram for gram, fats contain twice the calories of carbohydrates and protein, so a teaspoon of fat such as butter, margarine or oil will provide 37 calories while a teaspoon of a protein food like lean beef will provide around 10. A fatty diet is therefore far more energy dense than one rich in carbohydrates and proteins. That is, many more calories are packed into a small quantity of fatty foods than are contained in carbohydrates and proteins.

It's easy to monitor the amount of fats we take in when we can actually *see* them. These so-called 'visible fats' are things like butter, margarines and oils. They are all virtually 100 per cent pure fat and are very high in calories. Much more of a problem are the fats lurking in foods, and in some cases drinks, that are well disguised. Looking on the packets of foods often gives the game away. If fats, oils, margarine or butter appear high up on the list of ingredients, then it is sure to contain a fair amount of them as ingredients are listed in order of the quantity used, with whatever there is most of appearing first and whatever there is least of appearing last. There are many foods containing such hidden fats that, in theory, aren't a surprise. Biscuits and cakes, creamy foods and things that are fried are bound to be rich in fats. Sometimes the actual quantities they contain can be quite staggering though.

Hidden Fats in Foods

2 shortbread fingers	9 g (⅓ oz)
2 coconut cookies	5 g (⅕ oz)
2 lemon puffs	10 g (⅓ oz)
Original crunchy bar	7 g (¼ oz)
Cherry bakewell	7 g (¼ oz)
Apple pie	8 g (¼ oz)
Puff slice	12 g (½ oz)
Flapjack slice	6 g (⅕ oz)
Viennese whirl	13 g (½ oz)
Cheese and tomato pizza (200g)	20 g (¾ oz)
Pork pie	37 g (1⅓ oz)
Steak and kidney pie	22 g (¾ oz)
2 pork sausages	30 g (1 oz)
Cornish pasty	29 g (1 oz)
Sausage roll	16 g (½ oz)
Fish and chips	38 g (1⅓ oz)
Coleslaw (per 50 g/2 oz)	8 g (¼ oz)

Savoury snacks are an area to really watch. Most are based on potatoes or corn and are then fried. Both potato and corn are able to absorb large amounts of fats during frying, so will be literally dripping in calories.

Snack	Packet Size	Calories	Fat
Bombay mix	100 g (4 oz)	494	32 g (1 oz)
Potato crisps	30 g (1 oz)	160	11 g (⅓ oz)
Peanuts	25 g (1 oz)	143	12 g (½ oz)
Trail mix	100 g (4 oz)	495	31 g (1 oz)
Les mignons	100 g (4 oz)	515	35 g (1¼ oz)
Tortilla chips	100 g (4 oz)	490	25 g (1 oz)

Other foods to be aware of are those with added cheese. Cheese is an excellent source of protein and calcium. However, it is also high in fats, the amount varying depending on the type, so if cheese is sprinkled over something such as a pizza or jacket potato, the totals of fat and calories will shoot up.

Returning to the valve. This little muscular ring at the entrance to the stomach is susceptible to chemicals in food over and above just proteins and fats. Perhaps one of the most surprising of these is peppermint. It is fairly traditional to serve mints after a meal as they do aid digestion further down the tract. In those who are prone to gastric reflux, the best advice is to pass on them. The peppermint acts as a smooth muscle relaxant. When it comes into contact with the sphincter, therefore, it will cause it to relax and lose tone, making it easier for the stomach contents to leak back into the oesophagus.

Caffeine, found in coffee, tea and cola, has a similar effect, making the ritual of coffee and mints after a meal a complete nightmare for the refluxer. The amount of caffeine commonly found in just one or two cups of coffee has been shown to slightly relax the valve just 30 to 45 minutes after drinking it.

If the mints are coated in chocolate, this will truly seal your fate as chocolate is yet another substance that will relax the valve acting as the stomach's gatekeeper. The effect of chocolate on the valve may be due to its methylxanthine content. Methylxanthines are related to the caffeine family of substances. Drinking hot chocolate, even the reduced fat versions, before going to bed is also a habit best discouraged if heartburn is a problem.

Alcohol weakens the muscular valve, too, so, again, go easy, and a liqueur is the last the thing you need after a big meal.

Some evidence suggests that onions and garlic have adverse effects on valve tone, too, so it is worth testing the theory out and seeing if reducing them in the diet works for you.

Concentrated solutions of sugar or salt may directly irritate the oesophageal membranes that have already been damaged by reflux. This may explain why some fruit juices and tomato juice are poorly tolerated. The high sugar concentration may be more irritating than the acid content. Spicy foods can also have a direct, negative effect on the already damaged areas.

Action Plan

Heartburn due to reflux is painful and distressing and eventually will take the enjoyment out of eating and drinking. Reduce the risks of reflux by following the simple rules below.

Plan Your Meals

Make time for your meals, however little spare you have, by setting aside a calm 20 minutes to eat and drink. Eating on the hoof can be a false economy where time is concerned if following the meal you are then debilitated by uncomfortable refluxing.

One way of slowing down is to use a different method of eating to the one you normally use. Try chopsticks, for example. If you are not practised in using them, they will definitely slow you down, although, of course, this isn't very practical when you are out in restaurants or with friends.

Chew slowly. Start by training yourself to chew everything 40 times before swallowing. It has a remarkably calming effect and presents food to your stomach in a more digestible form.

Eat little and often. Plan your day so that you don't have any heavy meals at night time. If you get peckish in the evenings, then stick to light fruits or yogurts.

Avoid cigarette smoking, especially in the evening before going to bed, as this weakens the valve to the stomach.

Get the overall balance of your diet right by including the correct amounts of starchy carbohydrates, proteins, fats and sugars.

Drinks

As a rule, try to avoid coffee and strong tea, as well as hot chocolate and cola drinks. Decaffeinated versions of tea, coffee and cola can be found, but, still, go easy as they do contain some caffeine.

Alternatives include drinks such as Barley Cup and Caro, herb teas and herb-based soft drinks, such as Purdys and Aqua Libra, and you can't go wrong with straightforward still water.

Intakes of alcohol do need to be controlled and kept to a minimum because, as we have seen, it is able to loosen the stomach valve.

Gastritis

Spices contain volatile oils, which are also capable of physically irritating the stomach lining. This is a purely direct physical reaction, unlike the chain of events set in motion by caffeine production. Hot curries, chillies and chilli sauces used in Mexican and other foods and some drinks, like spicy tomato juices, Virgin and Bloody Marys are best avoided. A very hot chilli or curry dish that contains a blend of pungent spices can literally bore a hole in the stomach lining.

Foods to Eat

- dairy products, such as milk, milky drinks, yogurts, fromage frais, cottage cheese, custards and rice puddings
- foods rich in soluble fibre, which includes porridge oats and stewed apples and pears
- soft, non-acidic fruits, including melons, guavas, papayas and apricots – both dried and rehydrated
- Root vegetables, including potatoes, turnips and parsnips

Foods to Avoid

- spicy dishes, such as curries, if you are not used to them
- chillies in dishes and drinks

Drinks to Take

- skimmed milk-based drinks, using coffee and tea substitutes
- vegetable juices not based on tomato, such as carrot
- water

Drinks to Avoid

- fruit juices
- tomato juice
- coffee
- tea
- cola drinks

Burping and Belching

Burping and belching, like clothes and food, are subject to fashions and trends. Considered a sign of appreciation after a good meal back in Tudor times, burping after a dinner party nowadays would offend and embarrass the other people there. So, burping and belching are now largely consigned unceremoniously to the indigestion category as something we want to avoid.

Both long, hearty belches and short, sharp burps are, whatever your attitude towards them, a perfectly normal part of the digestive process, as they help to expel air that has collected in the stomach. While a baby is growing in the womb, the digestive tract is free from air. Once born, from the first inhalation of breath, the system gradually takes in air, especially when feeding, making it inevitable that the baby will need to burp.

When we need to burp, this indicates that quite a bit of air has accumulated in the stomach. This can produce symptoms varying from mild discomfort to quite unbearable cramping pain. Releasing the air from the stomach, up into the oesophagus and out of the mouth gives almost immediate relief.

Once again, eating habits, smoking and lifestyle all affect the quantity of air swallowed and produced. If air were water, straightforward swallowing involves taking down about a teaspoonful. Eating quickly, chatting, laughing, smoking and consuming carbonated drinks all increase the quantity of air swallowed and the necessity to bring it back up as burps or belches.

Dietary Advice

The advice for belching is very similar to that for bloating. It is especially important in this case to eat slowly and not to eat and talk at the same time as this encourages large amounts of air to be swallowed along with the food.

Chewing gum is also not recommended, and avoid carbonated drinks.

Eat and drink slowly, making time for both. Doing either quickly will lead to swallowing large amounts of air and so aggravate belching problems.

An infusion of ginger can help relieve the need to belch. Try pouring boiling water into a cup containing a teaspoon of freshly grated ginger root and leave the mixture to stand for five minutes before straining off the liquid and drinking it. Alternatively, you could try chewing a ginger biscuit.

If you don't suffer from reflux, sucking a strong peppermint may also help relieve the problem.

Gently rubbing the stomach can help dislodge any trapped wind in the stomach, as can bending down from the waist or taking gentle exercise.

Food Diaries

If you suffer regularly from belching, and, indeed, flatulence, dietary culprits can often be identified by keeping a food diary. This involves writing down everything you eat and drink over a five or seven-day period. It is necessary to record the times the food and drink were consumed and how you felt at the meal – whether it was rushed, whether you sat and had it quietly and so on. You also then need to record the time and severity of any symptoms that follow.

Over the course of a week, it should be possible to identify whether certain foods, drinks or situations are regularly precipitating the problem. It may seem like a chore, but this is a proven method of identifying causes of problems. For instance, a lot of people who suffer migraines complete such diaries to help identify trigger factors for their severe and debilitating headaches.

You can create your own food diary by buying a small notebook or just stapling a few sheets of paper together and creating a table set out like the following example.

Looking at this food diary, the information indicates that breakfast is not a problem. By mid-afternoon, however, the effect of lunch is showing up as a gassy, bloated feeling. This could have been due to rushing the food down and having a fizzy cola drink. If there were lots of beans in the chilli and it was very hot and spicy, this could have led to the bloating.

Food Diary

Date:

Food/drink	Amount	Time	Type of meal	Time taken to consume	Feelings	Symptoms
Toast	x 2	8 am	Small	10 mins	Rushed	None
Butter	1 tsp					
Jam	1 tsp					
Tea	cup					
Baked potato	x1	1 pm	Medium	15 mins	Rushed	None
Chilli sauce						
Cola	Glass					
Tea						
Bun	x1	3 pm	Snack	5 mins	Rushed	Gassy, bloated
Meat	Small	8 pm	Dinner	30 mins	Quiet	OK
Cabbage	2 tbsp					
Carrots	2 tbsp					
Potatoes	x 3					
Treacle tart	1 slice					
Cream	Dollop					
Coffee						
Tea	Cup	10 pm		10 mins	Quiet	Belching, full

The snack in the afternoon didn't cause problems, but dinner looks quite heavy and, later in the evening, resulted in a full feeling and belching. The cabbage may have caused the belching and the fatty, heavy dessert led to that uncomfortable fullness, which is a bad state to go to bed in.

It may have been better to have had a fish or low-fat cheese filling with the baked potato at lunchtime and a still drink instead of a fizzy one and to have left more time to eat it, too. For dinner, substituting a different green vegetable, such as spinach or broccoli, and following this with a lighter dessert, like baked apple with fromage frais, may have helped avoid the problem.

Gastric Ulcers

Ulcers can occur in the stomach, which account for about 20 per cent of all ulcers, or, much more commonly, in the duodenum, which make up the remaining 80 per cent.

Stomach, or gastric, ulcers must be taken seriously. They can be the next step on from gastritis, which is when local areas of the lining of the wall of the stomach are eroded. Unlike gastritis, ulcers don't just occur due to an overproduction of, or imbalances in, acid production. Gastric ulcers can be single or multiple, acute or chronic, large or small. They can appear, heal and leave you in peace then re-emerge again suddenly. The acid production is often normal or even reduced in people who suffer stomach ulcers, so the problem seems more likely to stem from the mucus not being able to withstand the normal acidic conditions in the stomach. This might be because it has been under constant attack from irritants, such as aspirin and alcohol.

Gastric ulcers can cause discomfort once in a while or can, at the other end of the spectrum, lead to excruciating pain if the ulcer perforates and penetrates into surrounding tissues or organs. Pain associated with stomach ulcers usually sets in around one to one and a half hours after eating.

There is no strong consensus on 'natural' causes of ulcers. They do seem, however, to run in families, occur in people with type O blood and in those who push themselves hard at work and often at play as well.

There is a growing consensus in the medical world that a large number of ulcers are caused by an infective agent, a bacteria called *Helicobacter pylori*. Work carried out in Australia by Dr Barry Marshall and his team of researchers revealed that, on average, *H. pylori* is present in 65 per cent of patients with stomach ulcers and 85 per cent with duodenal ulcers. However, *H. pylori* is present in the stomachs of many people who don't have ulcers, so the link between this bacteria and ulcers is not quite clear. It could be that people carrying *H. pylori* get ulcers by an unfortunate quirk of their biochemical make-up. If this is so, it would fit in with the observation that ulcers tend to affect members of the same family.

It is known that certain drugs used for arthritis – non-steroidal anti-inflammatory drugs (NSAIDs) – can, unfortunately, lead to perforation of the stomach wall, as can large, continued doses of aspirin.

Ultimately, drugs will probably be needed to heal the ulcer. However, diet and lifestyle can contribute to the relief of symptoms and help in the healing process.

Dietary Advice

The good news is that the old-fashioned diets of bland foods based on milk and milk puddings and strict dietary programmes have not been proven to be effective in the treatment and management of gastric ulcers, so there is no need to restrict yourself to these kinds of uninspiring choices.

For years, it was believed that milk somehow neutralized an 'acid stomach'. Tests have shown that milk has only a passing neutralizing effect on gastric acids and is actually rapidly followed by a rise in acidity. So, it seems that those who spent long periods on a bland diet of white fish, mashed potato and milky drinks did so in vain. Such a regimen *doesn't* help to heal ulcers.

There are some general guidelines which can be followed as part of a modern gastric diet:

- meals should be small, frequent and regular
- very hot or very cold foods should be avoided as they encourage air to be swallowed, which aggravates the problems
- fried foods should be avoided
- leave out any pickles, black pepper, vinegar, spices and mustard
- avoid tea, coffee, colas, cold remedies with caffeine and alcohol, which all stimulate acid production
- according to herbalists, liquorice has a soothing action on mucous membranes and is often given to help treat ulcers (it can be taken as a drink by pouring hot water over a liquorice root and allowing to simmer for 15 minutes).

While consumption of alcohol can rarely be identified as the cause of an ulcer, wine and drinks with 5 per cent or more alcohol are potent stimulants of gastric acid secretion and should therefore be avoided by those with ulcers.

Caffeine again rears its head. Like alcohol, most studies have revealed that while it doesn't *cause* ulcers, it can exacerbate pre-existing conditions. Tea has been shown to have a similar effect after just 200 ml has been consumed, which is just a couple of mugs.

B_6 is a vitamin found in meat, milk, potatoes and other vegetables. Some ulcer sufferers have been found to have low levels of this vitamin circulating in the blood. It has been suggested that supplementing with B_6 vitamin could help in the healing of ulcers. The same is true of observational studies on gastric ulcer patients who have taken vitamin C supplements.

Foods rich in vitamin C include all citrus fruits, such as oranges and grapefruits and their respective juices, berries, like strawberries, raspberries and blackberries, kiwi fruit, peppers including red, yellow and green, green leafy vegetables, sweet potatoes, parsley and, in smaller amounts, parsley and ordinary potatoes.

Modest supplements of both vitamins B$_6$ and C could be considered, but check with your doctor before taking them.

Some research has shown that when laser therapy was given to a group of people with gastric ulcers, it was more effective when given together with vitamin E supplements.

Vitamin E is found in good amounts in wheatgerm oil, and other vegetable oils, wholegrain cereals, eggs, dark green leafy vegetables, such as spinach and dark green cabbage, and sprouts. Avocados are also a good source, as are blackberries.

Taking zinc sulphate supplements has also been looked into and seems to have a degree of success in some people with gastric ulcers. Note, though, that it is easy to take too much zinc, so don't take this supplement without checking amounts with your doctor.

Oysters are the best, and unfortunately the most expensive, source of zinc. Red meat is the next best, however, with lean beef and lean pork boasting the highest amounts. Cheddar cheese is also rich in zinc, as are the dark meat from chicken, lentils, wholegrain cereals, rice and maize.

Work has also been carried out on the effect of essential fatty acids (EFAs) on gastric ulcers. Both those found in vegetable oils, such as sunflower, safflower and evening primrose, as well as those from oily fish, like salmon, tuna, mackerel, sardines, kippers and pilchards, have been indicated to have a positive effect.

It seems that the EFAs in the vegetable oils may enhance ulcer healing. The theory behind their role lies in the fact that EFAs are converted in the body into hormone-like substances known as prostaglandins. Various pieces of evidence indicate these prostaglandins may play a physiological role in protecting the gastric mucous membranes. Supplementing with EFAs in the form of evening primrose oil (Efamol) and fish oils may help protect against and treat ulcers.

There is some evidence that high-fibre diets may be of benefit – not in the healing process, but in delaying the time of another ulcer occurring. This is an area in which further study is needed, but, as a high-fibre diet is essentially a healthy way of eating and will help to provide the nutrients mentioned above, for example B_6, zinc and vitamins C and E, it is certainly worth following such a diet.

Foods rich in fibre include wholegrain breads, wholegrain cereals, like brown rice and pasta, and breakfast cereals such as bran flakes, All Bran, Weetabix, Shredded Wheat, porridge and muesli and granola. Pulses, vegetables and fruit are also good sources.

There is not enough proof from these research findings for dietitians to recommend particular strategies based on them to patients, but they are continuing areas of interest and more remains to be found out and confirmed.

5

The Small Intestine

After the stomach, the gut reverts to a tube shape, and this part of the digestive system is the small intestine. Only about 2.5 cm (1 in) wide, it's a staggering 2 m (2 yards) long. This great length of tubing is carefully arranged in the region we usually refer to as our stomach – the space below the ribcage. If the intestines were stretched out rather than being neatly folded as they are, we would be a very tall race.

The small intestine is where the bulk of the digestive process takes place. The stomach has mechanically turned the food and drink into the liquidy chyme described earlier, and between it and the mouth has already started chemically breaking down proteins, carbohydrates and fats. The small intestine, though, is sitting in wait with a complete army of enzymes to continue the job. It is here where proteins are broken down into their smallest form, amino acids, carbohydrates to simple sugars and fats to fatty acids and glycerol. It is here also where essential vitamins and minerals in foods are absorbed into the blood to be carried off to perform various functions around the body.

Under the microscope, the wall of the small intestine looks like grass blowing in the wind. This is because the wall is formed into very fine finger-like projections known as villi (see Figure 5). They are about a millimetre (less than ⅛ in) tall and feel velvety. Digested nutrients are absorbed through the wall of villi into little blood vessels which run inside them.

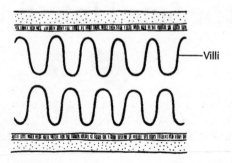

Figure 5 The villi on the walls of the small intestine.

The villi increase the absorbtive surface of the small intestine enormously – yet another space-saving device. It has been estimated that the entire absorptive surface these villi provide is equivalent to 200 sq. m (239 sq. yards). That is, the floor space of an average two-storey house. If there were no villi, the small intestine would have to be even longer than it already is.

Intestinal juices, which contain some of the necessary breakdown enzymes, are secreted from the walls of the intestine in quantities of 1 to 2 litres a day. They pour into the intestine when the chyme leaves the stomach and enters the duodenum.

Enzymes are also secreted directly from the intestinal walls and from the pancreas – an organ that sits alongside the intestine and also secretes some enzymes. The pancreas is vital for another reason. The chyme from the stomach is still acidic at this point and must be made neutral so that it doesn't damage the intestine wall. The pancreas pumps alkaline juices into the intestine to effect this neutralization.

In addition to enzymes, the intestine receives a secretion from the gallbladder – another small organ situated close by. The gallbladder squirts in bile, which is a rather unpleasant-looking yellowy green liquid. This happens when the intestine registers that the chyme from the stomach is particularly fatty after a fat-rich meal has been eaten. The hormone cholecystokinin (CCK) acts as the messenger, racing from the intestine to tell the gall-bladder to start firing. Bile is able to emulsify or homogenize fats. A good example of homogenization is homogenized milk, which has the fat evenly distributed throughout so that no cream line forms. This, essentially, is what bile does to fats in the intestine. It distributes them evenly, thus giving the fat-breaking enzymes a chance to get to work on them.

Food is moved down the tube by the muscles that surround it. They contract and relax rhythmically in a motion known as peristalsis (see Figure 6). These little waves of movement gradually push the contents forwards and backwards, offering them up to the villi to be absorbed.

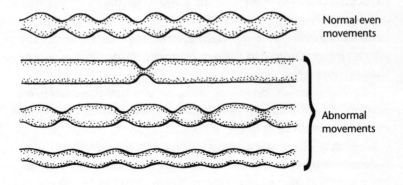

Normal even movements

Abnormal movements

Figure 6 Rhythmical movements – known as peristalsis – in the small intestine push the contents along.

The end of the small intestine is blocked off from the start of the final section of the system – the large intestine – by another valve. Nerves and hormones tell the valve to open to allow undigested material from the meal and bacteria to move on into the large intestine. The valve is important not so much for letting the material through, but for stopping contents of the large intestine creeping back into the small intestine.

The small intestine, like the stomach, is wired up to the brain via a huge number of nerves. Thus, any stress, anxiety or worries can again be transmitted to the system and affect its functioning in very significant ways.

Duodenal Ulcers

These are ulcers that develop in the very first part of the small intestine and seem, unlike stomach, or gastric ulcers, to be a result of overproduction of acid in the stomach. They can also develop as a result of the stomach emptying too much of its acidic contents into the duodenum in one go, and the duodenum having insufficient alkaline secretions present to neutralize them. The bacteria *H. pylori,* mentioned above, may play an important role in the development of duodenal as well as stomach ulcers.

Like gastric ulcers, duodenal ulcers occur when there has been erosion of the mucous membranes. They may be single or multiple, superficial or deep.

Duodenal ulcers seem to be strongly hereditary – probably because the overproduction of acid runs in families. They are far more common than stomach ulcers. The finger of blame can, once again, in part, be pointed at stress. This was seen clearly to be the case in London during the Second World War where the number of people with ulcers increased dramatically during the air raids. The theory goes that excessive nerve stimulation increased acid production, which led to duodenal ulcers developing. While air raids are a thing of the past, it's easy to see how the pressures of modern life could easily lead to a similar end result. Tight deadlines, frantic schedules, combining family responsibilities with work, bringing up children, financial and emotional worries, combined with other day-to-day problems can create untold stress.

Dietary Advice

Similar dietary guidelines apply for duodenal ulcers as stomach ulcers.

Researchers have tried treating duodenal ulcers with apple pectin (the substance in fruit that makes jam set). When patients were given around 12 mg a day, the pectin seemed to help prevent relapses. The researchers suggest that apple pectin could therefore be used as a form of treatment to help reduce the risk of recurring duodenal ulcers. This treatment is not widely used, however, and so should be talked through with your doctor.

A generally high-fibre diet may, as with stomach ulcers, help reduce the risk of further duodenal ulcers occurring. Research with patients who have duodenal ulcers has shown a dramatically lowered incidence of recurrence in those who follow such a diet, which, some researchers believe, could be because of the increased amount of chewing high-fibre diets require. The extra chewing means more saliva is produced. Saliva is, you will recall, alkaline. The increased flow of this alkaline fluid into the stomach helps lower stomach acidity and, thus, reduces the risk of irritation to the mucous membranes there. Whether or not this theory is true, a high-fibre diet has many other benefits with regard to problems with digestion and so is worth adopting anyway.

Continuously high alcohol intakes seem to cause more duodenal ulcers than gastric ones and so should be avoided wherever possible.

Tea and coffee should also be kept to a minimum so as to avoid encouraging extra acid to be secreted in the stomach.

To avoid developing or to recover from duodenal ulcers, you should follow a low-fat diet. Some fats are necessary as they contain vitamins A, D and E and EFAs. The ones that provide such nutrients are the vegetable and fish oils. Saturated animal fats – found in fatty cuts of meat, the skin of poultry, butter, full-cream dairy products and in manufactured products like pies, pastries, cakes, biscuits and so on – need to be cut right back, and the fats which are eaten need to come from vegetable oils, nuts and seeds and oily fish.

There could be a need for EFAs to be taken as supplements. It has been found that men suffering from duodenal ulcers have significantly lower amounts of the EFA linoleic acid in their abdominal walls than do healthy men. As the amount of linoleic acid stored in fat in the body reflects the amount that is eaten, it would seem that duodenal ulcer sufferers have a lower intake than non-sufferers. As mentioned under Gastric Ulcers, in Chapter 4, the linings of the mucous membranes may be protected by prostaglandins, substances made from linoleic acid. A good supplementary source of EFAs that the body can easily turn into prostaglandins is evening primrose oil.

Gallbladder Problems

When the gallbladder starts producing gallstones, eating can become a complete misery. Soon after indulging in a fatty meal or even just a fatty snack, a person with gallstones can experience severe flatulence along with gripping chest pains. So, what is the gallbladder and why does it cause symptoms of indigestion when it goes wrong?

The gallbladder sits alongside the intestine. It is a thin-walled, small, green, muscular sack or bag that, like a miniature version of the stomach, can expand and contract in size depending on the volume of its contents. It is around 10 cm (4 in) long and can hold between 30 and 50 ml (1 and 2 fl oz), which is about a third of a small yogurt pot. The gallbladder looks a bit like a two-tentacled octopus, with its rounded 'head' connected to both the liver and the top part of the small intestine by two different ducts or tubes.

The gallbladder's function is to store a thick, liquid substance called bile and to release it into the intestine when required. The liver makes the bile and sends it to the gallbladder via one of the ducts. It stays in the gallbladder until the hormone called CCK arrives on the scene, instructing it to shoot bile into the other duct, which leads into the intestine. CCK also has the effect of relaxing the valve located where the duct joins the intestine, thus allowing the bile in.

Bile has one main constituent that helps indigestion – bile salts. Bile salts help break down and emulsify fats in the intestine and distribute them evenly throughout the rest of the chyme. As mentioned earlier, this is a bit like what happens when milk is homogenized, when the creamy part is thoroughly mixed in with the watery part of the milk, making the fat and water homogenous.

The bile salts, therefore, physically separate the big globules of fat – eaten, for example, in the form of cheese, butter, margarine or ice-cream – breaking them down into millions of tiny fatty droplets.

Bile also contains, among other things, cholesterol and pigments. It is the pigment that gives our stools their characteristic colour. Without bile, they would look a grey white colour and also contain fatty streaks as, without bile, fats are not properly digested or absorbed into the body.

The hormone CCK, which, you remember, stimulates the gallbladder to release bile, is itself released when the contents of the stomach moving into the intestine are rich in fats.

Problems with the gallbladder occur when it makes gallstones from cholesterol. Bile salts normally keep levels of cholesterol at the correct level, but if there is too much cholesterol for the bile salts to deal with, then the cholesterol crystallizes, forming the so-called 'stones'. These sit in the gallbladder itself and/or in the duct, obstructing the flow of bile. When the gallbladder or duct contracts in response to a fatty meal, the sharp crystals dig into the walls and cause agonizing pain, which spreads throughout the right side of the chest region, causing severe indigestion.

Gallstones are known to be a complication associated with obesity. It is well worth shedding excess weight to help avoid developing them. Also, people who are overweight experience worse symptoms when they have gallstones than do their normal weight counterparts. In the late 1980s, 88,837 women aged between 34 and 59 years were selected for a study and followed up over a 4-year period. They completed detailed food and alcohol intake diaries and their weights were recorded. It was found that there was a link between diet and weight in that the more overweight the women, the more likely they were to develop gall-stones. One woman who was 41 and over 25 kg (about 4 stone/ 56 lb) overweight went on a 1,000 calories a day diet. Over 15 months, she lost 19 kg (3 stone/42 lb), during which period her gallstones disappeared. After 19 months, she was down to her ideal weight and her gallbladder was working properly.

It would seem sensible, judging from the picture you can build from this research, that getting down to or keeping to a normal bodyweight is a must to give your gallbladder a chance of working properly.

Gallstones can be surgically removed. It is also possible to dissolve the crystals. Nowadays, however, they are more likely to be treated by ultrasound vibrations, which pulverize, or lasers, which vaporize them.

Dietary Advice

A low-fat diet is often prescribed for people who suffer from gall-stones. Its effectiveness has not been completely tried and tested with enough clinical studies to know for certain whether or not it is truly effective. However, it does seem to make sense that if fatty foods stimulate the gallbladder to contract and deliver bile to the intestine, that a low-fat diet will reduce its activity and, thus, discomfort. Very often, it's a case of trial and error when working out just how much fat can be tolerated by an individual, and it is worth experimenting with.

Most people in the West eat diets with around 40 to 45 per cent of the total calories coming from fat. This needs to be reduced to 35 per cent for normal fit people. If you suffer from gallstones, you could try reducing your fat intake to more like the 30 per cent level to see if this helps improve symptoms. For a woman who eats about 2,000 calories a day, 30 per cent of this would be 600 calories. As 1 g of fat contains 9 calories, this would mean that she would need to keep the total grams of fat eaten in a day down to around 67 g (2½ oz). For a man eating a total of 2,550 calories a day, 30 per cent of this would be 765. This would translate into a daily total of 85 g (3½ oz) of fat.

For most people, meat and meat products, like sausages, beefburgers, meat pies and pasties, the spreading fats, like butter and margarine, cooking oils, full-fat milk and dairy products, such as cheeses, cream and full-fat yogurts, are the main sources of fat in the diet because they are eaten on a daily basis. Fats hidden within other foods, like savoury snacks, pastries, biscuits, cakes and puddings and other desserts, also add a considerable and increasing amount of fat to the diet and need to be carefully controlled when on a low-fat diet.

Over the last few years, there has been an enormous growth in the number of reduced and low-fat products appearing on the supermarket shelves, and these can help enormously when you are following a low-fat plan.

Skimmed milk is now readily available, as are reduced or virtually fat-free dairy products, including yogurts, fromage frais, cheeses, ready-made custards and milk puddings. There are also many low-fat and very low-fat spreads, although if you don't like any of them, just use the minimum amount of butter or a traditional margarine. Low-fat ready meals fill the freezer and chill cabinets, and all kinds of reduced-fat crisps, chips, sausages, burgers, dressings and even ice-creams are now on the market.

The following lists of foods – divided into very low-fat, low-fat, medium- and high- fat categories – can help guide you as to the good and bad foods. However, check before you buy because some reduced-fat products are still, compared to other foods, relatively quite fatty. Reduced-fat Cheddar, for example, is still a medium-fat food.

Very Low-fat Foods (less than 5 g per 100 g/⅛ oz per 4 oz)

- skimmed milk
- low-fat yogurt
- egg white
- cottage cheese
- turkey breast, skinless, grilled
- white fish, poached or steamed
- shellfish, steamed
- all vegetables, including potatoes, cooked without fat
- salad vegetables, without dressing
- beans, peas and lentils
- plain boiled sweets
- jam and honey
- sauces and pickles
- Marmite (yeast extract)
- bread
- pasta
- breakfast cereals

- crispbreads
- meringues
- jellies
- custard and rice pudding, made with skimmed milk
- fruits, fresh, frozen, canned

Low-fat Foods (5–10 g fat per 100 g/⅛–¼ oz per 4 oz)

- ham
- lean steak, grilled
- lean roast beef, leg pork, leg lamb, roast chicken, without skin
- kidneys, grilled
- pilchards
- roast potatoes
- oven chips
- cream and thick soups
- muesli (granola)
- Ready Brek
- soft rolls
- currant buns
- sponge, such as Swiss roll
- trifle
- ice-cream
- apple crumble

Medium-fat Foods
(containing 10–20 g fat per 100 g/¼–¾ oz per 4 oz)

- full-fat yogurt
- boiled eggs
- Feta cheese
- curd cheese
- reduced-fat Cheddar
- lean back bacon, grilled
- rump steak, fried
- mince, stewed
- lean lamb and pork chops
- chicken, roasted, with skin
- beefburgers, hamburgers
- livers, fried
- cod in batter, fried
- salmon, tinned
- sardines
- fish fingers
- scampi, fried
- thick-cut chips/french fries
- olives
- Mars bar
- toffees
- cream crackers
- rich tea biscuits
- oatcakes
- ginger nuts

- wafers
- rock and madeira cakes
- doughnuts
- scones
- fruit cakes
- pancakes
- sponge pudding
- fruit pies
- lemon meringue pie

High-fat Foods
(containing more than 20 g fat per 100 g/¾ oz per 4 oz)

- butter
- margarine
- cream, all types
- oils, all types
- mayonnaise, including low-fat varieties
- low-fat spreads
- salad cream, including low-fat varieties
- peanut butter
- eggs, scrambled and fried
- Scotch eggs
- Stilton
- cream cheeses
- Cheddar, Cheshire
- Parmesan
- Edam

- cheese spreads
- quiche
- Welsh rarebit
- streaky bacon, fried
- lamb and pork chops, with fat
- roast duck, with skin and fat
- liver pâté
- luncheon meat
- pork sausages
- sausage rolls
- pork pies
- pasties and meat pies
- taramasalata
- whitebait, fried
- chips (french fries), deep-fried
- crisps (potato chips), normal and low-fat varieties
- avocados
- soya beans
- nuts
- milk chocolate
- chocolate biscuits
- filled wafers
- custard creams
- shortbread
- pastry, all types
- Victoria sponge cake
- cream cakes

- pies
- cheesecakes

As to other pieces of advice, interestingly it has also been shown that women who skipped breakfast or only had coffee at the start of the day had a greater incidence of gallstones than did those who ate breakfast. So, taking breakfast may help prevent gallstones occurring.

In addition, it has been suggested and observed that frequent consumption of smoked foods also seems to encourage the formation of gallstones. Commonly consumed smoked foods include bacon and smoked mackerel.

The good news, though, is that a moderate intake of alcohol may actually help to reduce the incidence of gallstones.

Cholesterol in the Diet

It is commonly thought that when foods known to be rich in cholesterol, such as egg yolks, fish roe and shellfish are eaten, the cholesterol levels in the blood will rise once the foods have been digested. In fact, scientists have never been able to show that blood cholesterol rises after eating such foods. Most of the cholesterol in the blood is made by the body itself. Levels of cholesterol rise if the diet is rich in saturated fats, found in animal fats, dairy products, coconut oil and coconut cream and foods containing these fats.

The incidence of gallstones in France, India, Japan, Portugal, South Africa, Sweden and Uganda was studied back in 1978 and the results showed that in those countries where total calories and fat intakes were lower and vegetable intakes higher, few people had gallstones. After the Second World War, the incidence of gallstones increased in France over a 20-year period. The increases occurred as the diets increased in total calories and fats.

Studies that compared vegetarian women with non-vegetarian women have revealed that, as a group, vegetarian women have less than half the incidence of gallstones of their meat-eating sisters. The researchers carrying out the study believed that this finding could be attributed to the fact that the vegetarians ate less fat and more fibre.

From this it is clear that to help reduce cholesterol levels in the body, it is necessary to keep consumption of saturated fats well down. Eating foods rich in so-called 'soluble fibre' found in, for example, pulses, apples and oats, helps keep cholesterol levels down too.

Nausea

Most of us assume that nausea starts in the stomach. While this can happen, queasy feelings often in fact start in the duodenum due to local disturbances to its lining such as inflammation or ulceration. Messages are sent from the nerves in this upper part of the small intestine to the brain, which in turn feeds them back to the stomach. The distressing sensation it creates often leads to vomiting. Vomiting unsettles the peace of the tract, making the throat sore and leaving the mouth very acidic. It is important to try to calm the system by taking some rest and trying to drink some water to keep your fluid levels up.

Food Intolerances

Some people are born with and others develop intolerances to certain foods. These are not allergic reactions which involve the immune system, but are reproducible, unpleasant, non-psychological reactions to a specific food or food ingredient. It seems that the small intestine is particularly vulnerable to certain of these which, if not corrected, can cause symptoms which range from the uncomfortable to the potentially life threatening. For a calm and cleansed digestive tract, intolerances need to be diagnosed nearest the time of their onset as possible so that offending foods can be removed and order restored as quickly as possible.

Lactose Intolerance

Lactose is the sugar found in milk. It is known as a disaccharide or double sugar because it consists of the two single sugars glucose and galactose which are joined together. Lactose cannot be absorbed across the intestinal wall and into the blood until it has been broken down into glucose and galactose by the enzyme lactase, which sits in the wall.

A lack of the enzyme lactase gives rise to lactose intolerance – that is, the inability to break down lactose. This means the lactose passes undigested from the small intestine into the large intestine. Bacteria in the large intestine start fermenting the lactose, producing gases and irritating acids. These by-products of lactose fermentation lead to bloating, abdominal cramps and terrible wind. It is believed that just 2 g (⅛ oz) of lactose can lead to the production of 1,400 ml (50 fl oz) of hydrogen gas. One lactose-intolerant man was once recorded to have passed wind 141 times after consuming two pints of milk, a feat which made it into the *Guinness Book of Records*. The presence of lactose in the large intestine also has the effect of pulling in water and sugar from the surrounding blood vessels, which leads to profuse diarrhoea.

Lactose intolerance is usually an inherited problem. All newborn babies have enough lactase to cope with lactose in breastmilk or that found in infant formulas. After weaning, however, lactase activity decreases in all mammals, including humans. Lactase levels usually drop between the ages of two and five, and drop further in some than others. A child may start having symptoms of intolerance as late as when they first go to school.

In many parts of the world, entire races have very low levels of the lactase enzyme and thus cannot tolerate milk and dairy products. Many Asians, Native Americans and Japanese are in this position. Lactose intolerance can also start in later life, developing, for example, following intestinal infections, gastric surgery or a course of antibiotics or anti-inflammatory medication.

Usually the intolerance to milk's sugar is not absolute, meaning that the child or adult can cope with small amounts of dairy foods on a daily basis. Cheese and yogurt do not have high concentrations of lactose and are sometimes better tolerated as, fortunately, is chocolate.

Once diagnosed by your doctor, it is advisable to see a dietitian and work out a lactose-free diet for a specific period of time. Gradually, under his or her guidance, it is possible to reintroduce some milk products to assess how much, if any, can be tolerated. Since dairy products are such a valuable source of calcium, especially for the growing child, it is crucial that other sources of this essential mineral are consumed on a regular basis to ensure optimum bone mass is achieved and maintained. This requires a degree of dedication to the cause, but is well worth it for future health. Today it is also possible to buy calcium-enriched soya milk which is a very useful alternative.

Calcium-rich Foods

Foods	Mg of calcium per 100 g (4 oz) of food
Tahini	680
Sesame seeds	670
Tofu	510
Spinach	170
Sunflower seeds	110
Ready-to-eat apricots	73
Kidney beans	71
Peanuts	60
Peanut butter	37

Some people are intolerant to the proteins in milk and not the lactose. They would need to avoid the following foods:

all foods containing milk, cheese, butter, margarine, cream, cheese, yogurt, skimmed milk powder, non-fat milk solids, caseinates, whey, lactalbumin and lactose

biscuits (cookies)

breads, buns and bread mixes

breakfast cereals

cakes and cake mixes

flavoured crisps (potato chips)

gravy mixes

malted drinks

puddings and mixes, ice cream, custard, instant whips

sauces and cream soups

sausages and batters

sweets such as chocolate, fudge, toffee.

A full and comprehensive list of lactose- and milk protein-free foods is available from your local registered dietitian. Recognizing and dealing with milk intolerances is crucial to the settled functioning of the digestive system.

Gluten Intolerance

Coeliac disease is the condition which arises when an individual's small intestine lining is damaged by gluten, the protein found in wheat and rye, and by similar proteins found in barley and possibly oats. The long finger-like projections called villi (see page 40) which make up the wall of the small intestine become flattened when a person is intolerant to gluten, which means the surface area of this part of the digestive system is drastically reduced. This in turn leads to food speeding through without having a chance to be broken down and absorbed. Weight loss inevitably follows and the stools become either large, pale and with an offensive smell, or become loose, later developing into diarrhoea. Vomiting may also occur.

In children, a normal baby who is weaned onto foods containing gluten will start by refusing foods and then begin to lose weight. The child will become listless, and the stools change as described. The abdomen will swell, developing into what appears to be a pot belly.

In adults, the classic symptoms of indigestion can be the first signs of gluten intolerance. These could be anything from abdominal fullness and discomfort in the stomach region to diarrhoea, pain, vomiting and terrible tiredness. The changes to the stools may be a tell-tale sign, as they become pale, bulky and dreadfully smelly due to fat not being absorbed by the flattened intestinal walls and therefore remaining in the faeces.

Around one person in 1,850 is believed to have this intolerance to gluten in the UK, and although it runs in families the disease is not actually inherited. Quite what causes a person to become gluten-intolerant is still not really understood. Explanations have ranged from the gluten being intrinsically toxic to certain people because they lack a detoxifying enzyme, to the disease being an allergic reaction by the gut wall to the gluten. Neither theory really explains why it strikes a wide range of ages, or why different symptoms are experienced by different people.

Diagnosis, however, is crucial if digestive health is to be restored. This can only be done by a specialist doctor who takes a sample of the small intestine and studies it under the microscope to see if the villi are flattened.

Treatment for coeliac disease is to avoid gluten in the diet as much as possible. There are two main sources. The obvious sources are foods made from wheat flour or which contain barley or oats – bread, cereals, cakes, biscuits, pies and pastries, for example. Second, there are the less obvious sources. These are manufactured or processed foods that contain any of these cereals as fillers, thickeners, for bulking up and so on. They may be in the form of gluten, wheat starch, rusk or hydrolysed vegetable protein of wheat origin. They are added to the most unlikely things, such as sweets, as well as slightly more obvious ones, such as white sauces in boil-in-the-bag cod in parsley sauce and tinned foods like chicken in sauce.

Gluten-containing foods to avoid	Gluten-free alternatives
Cereals and cereal products	
Wheat, wholemeal, wholewheat and wheatmeal flours. Bran, barley, rye, rye flour, pasta and semolina.	Arrowroot, buckwheat, corn cornflour, maize and maize flour. Gluten-free flour, potato flour, rice and rice flour. Sago, soya and soya flour. Tapioca.

Cereals made from wheat, barley or rye, such as muesli, Shredded Wheat, Sugar Puffs and Weetabix. Baked products made from wheat, barley, rye flour, suet and semolina.

Rice Krispies and cornflakes.

Gluten-free baked biscuits, (cookies) bread, cakes and gluten-free pasta.

Crispbreads and starch-reduced bread and rolls. Ice-cream wafers and cones, plus Communion wafers.

Milk and milk products

Artificial cream containing flour. Yogurt containing muesli/granola.

Cheese spreads containing flour, which many do – check the labels.

Fresh, dried, condensed, evaporated, skimmed, sterilized. Fresh or tinned cream. Most yogurts. Cheddar, curd and cream cheeses.

Egg dishes

Eggs cooked with flour, such as Scotch eggs, eggs with white sauces. Quiches and egg flans.

Cooked without breadcrumbs and sauces.

Fats and oils

Suet contains flour.

All butters, margarines, oils, lard and dripping.

Meat and fish

Savoury pies and puddings made with flour. Any meat or fish with stuffings, breadcrumbs or suet. Sausages and burgers with bread-crumbs or rusk (check the

Plain meat and fish. Plain tinned fish. Check packaging of burgers and pre-packed meat – some are gluten-free.

packaging). Battered and crumbed fish, like fish fingers and fishcakes.

Vegetables, fruits and nuts

Tinned vegetables in sauces, such as creamed mushrooms. Potato croquettes. TVP containing wheat.

Fresh, tinned, cooked, dried and frozen, pulses and soya. Some baked beans – check the labels.

Fruit in fruit pies, crumbles and cakes.

Fresh, cooked, tinned, dried and frozen.

Nuts in cooked products and crackers and dry-roasted nuts.

Fresh, plain, salted.

Jams, sweets and desserts

Sweets containing or rolled in flour.Smarties, marshmallows, liquorice and Twix.

Sugar, glucose, jam, honey, marmalade, treacle, molasses, some mincemeat – check the label. Plain ice lollies/pops.

Puddings and desserts with flour, breadcrumbs and suet, such as pies crumbles and summer puddings. Ice-cream cones and wafers.

Jellies and milk puddings made from permitted cereals.
Check the labels of ice-cream and instant desserts as some are gluten-free. Not semolina.

Drinks

Barley-based instant coffee, barley-flavoured drinks. Bengers, malted drinks, such as Horlicks. Home-brewed beer, cloudy real ale and hot drinks from vending machines.

Tea, pure, instant or fresh ground coffee, cocoa, fizzy drinks, squashes and cordials, fresh fruit juices, wines, spirits, beer and lagers.

Soups, sauces and seasonings

Soups thickened with the cereals wheat, barley, rye or pasta. Bisto.	Home-made soups with suitable thickeners. Certain brands of tinned and dried soups. Certain gravy brownings. Check the packaging.
Some peppers, ready-mixed spices and curry powders.	Fresh peppers and herbs. Check the labels on other seasonings, mustards and powders.

Note: Beware that some medicines contain gluten, so check with the pharmacist or your doctor before taking anything if you are unsure.

Wheat Intolerance

In some cases, people are sensitive to wheat and wheat-containing foods, but when tested for coeliac disease are clearly not intolerant to gluten. While they must avoid wheat and wheat-containing foods, they are able to eat oats and barley. People sensitive to wheat are often those who eat a lot of it in breakfast cereals, pasta and bread. Wheat and other cereal staple crops were only introduced into our diets around 10,000 years ago (a blink of an eye in evolutionary terms), and it is believed that is why the problem is so common. Many people have not evolved the necessary digestive equipment to deal with the increasingly large quantities we throw at it on a daily basis.

With the help of a dietitian, the following foods need to be eliminated on a wheat-free diet:

some drinking chocolates and Horlicks

biscuits/cookies

cakes

bread – all types

breakfast cereals made from wheat

some cheese spreads, processed cheese and packet suet

some tinned fish and fish paste plus fish cooked in batter, breadcrumbs or a sauce

flours and cereals including wheatgerm, semolina, pasta and noodles

some canned meats and many ready meals, pies, sausage rolls, meat paste, paté and sausages

pastry

puddings (check the labels)

soups.

In addition, always check labels for the words 'wheat starch', 'edible' or 'modified starch', 'cereal filler', 'bran', 'rusk', 'cereal binder' or 'cereal protein'.

Fructose Intolerance

Rather like lactose intolerance, some people cannot cope with the fruit sugar fructose. Fructose is a single sugar found in fruits, and attached to glucose in table sugar. Thus all fruits and foods containing ordinary sugar need to be avoided. Fortunately, children born with fructose intolerance soon develop an innate and strong dislike of anything sweet-tasting, so they remain well as long as they are not forced to eat such foods. Since fruit and fruit juices must be avoided, it is important to ensure children get plenty of vegetables which supply the body with vitamin C, such as red, green, yellow and orange peppers, potatoes, sweet potatoes and, if you can persuade them, dark green leafy vegetables like spinach, broccoli and cabbage.

— 6 —
The Large Intestine

This section of the digestive tract is called 'large' because of its diameter rather than its length. It is half a metre (1½ feet) shorter than the small intestine and considerably fatter. Two main functions of the large intestine are to absorb water from indigestible food residues and to eliminate them from the body as semi-solid faeces (see Figure 7).

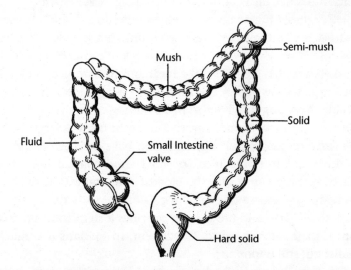

Figure 7 The semi-fluid contents of the small intestine are gradually turned into solids in the large intestine.

The large intestine is divided into five sections:

1. caecum
2. appendix
3. colon
4. rectum
5. anal canal.

Most of the main nutrients from food and drink have been absorbed once they reach the large intestine, so there is no reason to have all the little villi found on the surface of the small intestine. The surface is therefore flatter.

Although it is not having to secrete enzymes to break down nutrients like the small intestine, it would be wrong to give the impression that the large intestine is just a waste-processing plant. There are many, many metabolic processes taking place here which influence the health of the overall digestive system.

For example it actually synthesizes vitamin K, which is then absorbed across the large intestine's lining into the bloodstream. This role is vital since most of us eat insufficient vitamin K in our diets and it is crucial for the mechanisms involved in blood-clotting as well as energy metabolism. The large intestine is also capable of making the vitamins B_{12}, B_1 and B_2.

In addition to synthesizing certain vitamins, the large intestine converts sugars and starches which have not been absorbed by the small intestine into so-called short-chain fatty acids, which then cross over into the bloodstream and can be used by the body as a source of energy (or calories). In herbivores this short-chain fatty acid production provides a significant proportion of their calories, up to 22 per cent. In humans it is much smaller but still important.

The large intestine is also very much involved with water balance in the body. It receives large amounts of water from the small intestine, and an astonishing 7 litres (nearly 8 gallons) can be absorbed from it by the bloodstream in just 24 hours.

The large intestine is also home to millions and millions of bacteria and yeast, known as the gut flora. The flora feed on the remains of our meals, and on the whole are harmless. In fact, many are essential to the well-being of the gut. In a healthy person the gut flora get along just fine and create a balanced community. They literally cover the whole surface of the colon, many helping to prevent disease-causing bacteria from invading and taking over.

At certain times this finely balanced ecosystem may be disturbed, for example during a bout of food poisoning or through long-term use of antibiotics. Abnormalities in gut flora have been discovered in people suffering from Irritable Bowel Syndrome (see page 73), *Candida* overgrowth (see page 81) and similar diseases.

The large intestine does not move anything like as quickly as the small intestine and stomach. In fact, it can be rather like a lazy lizard basking in the sun, making the odd slow shuffling movement every half hour or so. By means of such movements, the residues of digestion are gradually shoved on round the colon until they reach the rectum. At this point nerves tell the rectum to contract and the valve to the anal canal opens. Once faeces enter the rectum, messages are sent to the brain and we then consciously decide whether or not to open the final valve of the whole system, the external anal valve, to allow expulsion of the stools.

The contents of the faeces, the exact components of the gut flora and the speed at which waste moves through the large intestine can all be significantly influenced by the food we eat. The overall health of this part of the digestive system is also intimately connected to our emotional well-being. Most of us will have experienced 'intestinal hurry' due to stress or fear at some time in our lives. Cleansing of the large intestine is possible through careful dietary choices and a thoughtful long-term approach to choices of foods and drinks.

Constipation

Constipation is, as anyone who has suffered will tell you, a pain in the 'you know where'. It results in a delaying of the time waste material travels down the large intestine to finally be passed as stools. The stools which do finally come out usually do so with a struggle, and tend to be hard and dry.

This troublesome condition which leads to a slowing down of transit times makes it easier for potential disease-causing organisms to take hold. The faster the waste passes through the large intestine, the more chance there is of nasties whizzing through it and leaving the body before they have had a chance to cause any damage. Avoiding constipation thus helps to keep the colon clean.

To know how to avoid constipation, you first need to know what causes it. There are several main reasons for the problem developing. One is simply ignoring your body when it is trying to tell you it is time to go to the loo. Sometimes this is completely understandable. Few people feel comfortable 'going' in someone else's home, in public loos and perhaps at work or when visiting relatives. The trouble is, putting off the call of nature because it's inconvenient makes the whole mechanism less sensitive and you trigger a vicious circle.

Another main cause of constipation is the formation of small faeces due to a diet which is low in fibrous wholegrain foods, vegetables and fruits. Emotions can also play a role, with depression often sparking off bouts of constipation. Pregnant women often fall foul of this complaint, due partly to the weight of the foetus pushing the uterus down onto the colon, which seems to delay bowel movements, and partly because of extra levels of the hormone progesterone, which slows colonic contractions down. The elderly can also be prone to constipation, as the nerves which feed the colon and which control its movements become less able to process the brain's messages telling them they need to go.

Higher rates of colonic cancer are associated with people whose transit times (the time it takes for waste from food to appear in the stools) are slow. It is thought that these slow transit times give potentially cancer-causing substances more time to latch on the colon wall. The faster the waste material moves through the colon, the more diluted these carcinogens become and the less time they have to establish themselves.

Transit times can be speeded up by increasing the bulk of the stool, which in turn increases the speed of transit. This is achieved by eating a diet rich in fibre and drinking plenty of fluids – which needs to be combined with making time to go the loo each day and tackling any underlying emotional problems.

Eating more fibre has other advantages when it comes to preventing cancer of the colon. The bacteria of gut use fibre and starches which have not been digested in the small intestine as food. In metabolizing the fibre they produce acids which lower the pH of the gut. This acidic environment is believed to decrease the activity of potential toxins. Not only this, the tannins, phytates and flavanoids found in wholegrain foods, fruits and vegetables bind to carcinogens, rendering them harmless.

Dietary Advice

Increasing the physical bulk of the faeces is one way in which to help overcome or avoid constipation. Diets rich in fruits, vegetables and wholegrain cereals provide the body with plenty of insoluble fibre. In the UK, the current average intake of fibre is around 12 g (about ¼ oz) a day – 6 g (about ⅛ oz) less than the recommended 18 g (about ¾ oz). The effect of diet on the faeces and how long they take to travel through the gut was shown by the research work carried out in the 1970s by a well-known fibre research expert, Professor Dennis Burkett.

He found that in the group of people from the UK who ate a typical British diet with lots of refined carbohydrates and therefore not much fibre, the food took around 83 hours to travel through the entire gut. The daily weight of the stools each person produced was, on average, 104 g (about 4 oz).

On the other hand, a group of Ugandan villagers who lived on an entirely unrefined diet containing a lot of fibre had transit times of 36 hours and produced 470 g (1 lb) of stools each a day.

Interestingly, he found that vegetarians in the UK who ate a mixed diet, some of which was unrefined, halved the transit time of their omniverous counterparts and more than doubled their stool weights.

There seems to be a very clear relationship between the composition of the diet and the speed with which the food moves through the gut. Soft, voluminous stools are much easier to pass and help to reduce problems further up the tract. Straining to pass stools over long periods, can, for example, exert pressure higher up in the digestive tract. It can cause pressure all the way back in the stomach and force the top stomach valve open, allowing its acidic contents to reflux back up into the gullet, causing heartburn and inflammation of the oesophagus. Also, such back pressure can affect the diaphragm and eventually lead to a hiatus hernia, which in turn pushes up the stomach and also causes gastric reflux.

A high-fibre diet is generally a healthy way of eating and also helps avoid constipation, but always check with your doctor that there is no underlying cause of constipation in your case and seek his or her approval regarding your going on a high-bulk diet.

Easy Steps Towards a High-fibre Diet

Always use wholegrain cereals where possible. This means wholemeal bread – not 'brown', but 100 per cent wholemeal. If you cannot tolerate this, try some of the white loaves with added fibre. Brown pasta and brown rice should be used instead of white. If this is unpalatable, try a half-white, half-brown mix. Eat 100 per cent wholewheat breakfast cereals, too, such as bran flakes, Shreddies, All Bran, Weetabix, Shredded Wheat or porridge.

The carbohydrate part of meals should be the central part, with other foods being added to this. Have, for example, a large serving of potatoes, rice or pasta and add to this a smaller portion of protein, such as meat, poultry, fish, eggs, cheese or pulses and nuts. This combination then needs to be accompanied by a large portion of vegetables, salad and/or fruit.

One crucial point to remember, however, is that all this will be in vain – and, indeed, have the opposite effect and clog you up – if it is not taken along with plenty of fluids. At least eight cups or glasses of fluid are needed a day in tandem with this highly unrefined diet to ensure that the stools will be soft and easy to pass. Cups of tea and coffee, juices and squashes all count towards this total eight. If you have a high-fibre diet and consume insufficient fluids, your stools end up looking and feeling like a cooked sausage that has been allowed to cool overnight. In other words, hard and difficult to pass, which is the opposite of what you want.

Diarrhoea

True diarrhoea is the frequent passing of loose or watery, unformed stools. It may happen suddenly and just occur once in a while or be a problem that continues over a period of time. Diarrhoea happens as a result of a problem in the small and/or large intestine.

The powerful effect of the nervous system on the gut has been mentioned several times so far, and diarrhoea is one of those symptoms everyone can associate with nerves. Pre-exam worries, big decisions, life-changing events, all are more than enough to trigger overactivity of neuromuscular connections, which speeds up peristalsis (the pulsating movement) of the intestinal walls and increases secretions, causing food and water to charge full-speed through the small and large intestines almost undigested.

Diarrhoea can also be the result of irritation or inflammation of the mucous membrane of the bowel by bacterial, viral, protozoal, chemical or physical agents. Diseases such as Crohn's disease and ulcerative colitis, as well as problems like gastroenteritis, also lead to frequent bouts of diarrhoea, which are hard to treat.

Obviously, it will be necessary to consult your doctor and find out the cause of the diarrhoea. If it *is* an on-going problem associated with a condition such as Crohn's or irritable bowel disease, solutions can be sought on an individual basis. If certain foods trigger it off, the intolerance needs to be investigated and identified with the help of a doctor. People often simply then avoid eating foods that tend to trigger off attacks.

Self-inflicted diarrhoea can occur where there is laxative abuse.

Whatever the cause, when sudden and large amounts of very loose stools are passed, above 1,000 g (2¼ lbs)a day, as well as water, huge amounts of water, sodium and potassium are lost, more than can be made up by eating and drinking normally. It is essential that the lost salts and water are replaced to prevent dehydration. If they are not, then irritability, fatigue, drowsiness, muscle cramps, thirst, loss of appetite, nausea, headache and faintness soon follow. A home remedy to replace the fluids and salts can be made up by taking 150 ml (¼ pint) boiling water and dissolving in this ½ teaspoon of salt and 4 heaped teaspoons of sugar. Add 150 ml (¼ pint) of fresh orange juice and then make up to 500 ml (17 fl oz) with water. This should be given in small quantities and at frequent intervals. Alternatively, commercial preparations such as Dioralyte can be used and are available from pharmacists.

It is vital that severe diarrhoea is investigated by your doctor if it persists.

Dietary Advice

As a rule, a bulky diet – in other words, a high-fibre diet – can, surprisingly, often be of help at such times. Instead of aggravating the system and rushing gut contents through at even greater speed, it can help bind the stools up a bit, making them bulkier and therefore slowing them down.

Irritable Bowel Syndrome

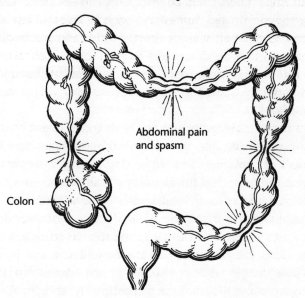

Figure 8 The large intestine of an IBS sufferer.

IBS has been identified as being related, in some women, to the pre-menstrual time of the month, and it is also often said to be brought on by stress, major surgery such as a hysterectomy, or the long-term use of antibiotics.

The one common link between all IBS sufferers, though, is that no physical ailment, such as Crohn's disease, ulcerative colitis, diverticulitis or cancer, can be identified. A great deal of specialist hospital time and equipment is necessary to eliminate all these other possible causes of the symptoms. Only after all the examinations have been carried out on the gut, and no such underlying cause can be detected, can a true diagnosis of IBS be made.

Defining what is normal for the bowels has always been a moot point. Some people can pass stools twice a day and think it is normal, while others could go three days and not consider themselves to be constipated. Some may always feel bloated after eating and consider it to be just a side-effect of eating and drinking, while others may find it uncomfortable enough to seek help. The incidence of IBS symptoms could in fact be even higher than the figures currently quoted as some sufferers may well never seek help or advice.

IBS is not a single entity and can be linked to many situations. Stress from, for example, divorce, moving house, losing a job or the death of someone close, hyperventilation, musculoskeletal problems and hormonal imbalances have all been cited as causes. That there are so many potential causes means that there is not one single effective treatment. Some doctors prescribe antispasmodic drugs, others bulking agents and some even tranquillizers. Dietary advice can also be helpful to some sufferers.

IBS provides yet another example of just how intimately the gut's reactions and the emotions can be linked. Taking time out for yourself to enjoy relaxation such as swimming, sitting in a sauna or steam room, having a massage, going to yoga or Pilates classes or simply taking a peaceful walk should all be considered alongside any dietary modifications you might consider.

Dietary Advice

Those who have specific symptoms of abdominal distension and wind may find that cutting out vegetables of the brassica family, such as cabbage, Brussels sprouts and broccoli, and pulses, such as red kidney, baked and black-eyed beans, as well as lentils, peas and chickpeas, and apples, grapes and raisins may help.

In the past, high-fibre diets have been recommended for IBS sufferers. Additions of up to 7 g (about ¼ oz) a day of wheat bran has, for example, been suggested for people who are suffering constipation as a result of IBS. Today, however, there is a movement away from bran, in recognition of the fact that intolerances to certain foods could be more to blame.

In order to detect which foods may be causing a specific person's problems, an exclusion diet needs to be followed. Research has proven that this has been effective in treating between 48 and 67 per cent of IBS patients. The exclusion diet developed in Cambridge at Addenbrookes Hospital is based on the plan set out below, but note that any kind of exclusion diet should only be undertaken with the permission of your GP and the guidance of a dietitian. This is necessary because it is not just a case of leaving out certain foods. It has to be done in a structured way and one that will provide meaningful results. The diet followed during the exclusion period and any diet prescribed afterwards for maintenance must be nutritionally adequate for the person concerned and this needs to be worked out with a qualified dietician.

Foods	Not Allowed	Allowed
Meat	Preserved meats, bacon, sausages	All other meats
Fish	Smoked fish, shellfish	White fish
Vegetables	Potatoes, onions, sweetcorn	All other vegetables
Fruit	Citrus fruits	All other fruit
Cereals	Wheat, barley, oats, corn, rye	Rice, tapioca, millet, buckwheat
Oils	Corn oil, vegetable oil	Sunflower, soya, safflower, olive oils
Dairy	Cows' and goat's milk, butter margarines, yogurts, cheese, eggs	Soya milk, milk-free margarine
Beverages	Tea, coffee, fruit squashes, grapefruit juice, alcohol, tap water	Herbal teas, apple, pineapple, tomato juices, mineral water
Other	Chocolate, yeast, vinegar, preservatives	Carob, salt, herbs, spices, sugar, honey

This is followed for two weeks and then the symptoms are reassessed. This needs to be done by your doctor. If there has been no improvement, then the person will be advised to return to their normal diet. If symptoms have cleared, however, the foods that were excluded are reintroduced, one at a time at two-day intervals in the following order:

● tap water

● potatoes

● cows' milk

● yeast

● tea

- rye
- butter
- onions
- eggs
- oats
- coffee
- chocolate
- barley
- citrus fruits
- corn
- cheese
- white wine
- shellfish
- yogurt
- vinegar
- wheat
- nuts
- preservatives.

When following such a plan, you need to keep a really close check on your symptoms and write them down on a daily basis.

Just to reinforce the point made above, though, it is vital that this kind of food exclusion diet is followed under the supervision of your doctor and a dietitian, who can ensure that the diet is kept to and that the food eaten is sufficiently rich in nutrients for your personal requirements to avoid any adverse effects of the exclusion.

After the results of the exclusion period and reintroduction of foods are known, how you should mix the foods that have been found to be well tolerated will also need to be worked out with your health-care provider to make sure that your diet will be providing all the necessary nutrients to maintain good health. It's no good having a diet that relieves the symptoms of IBS but is deficient in essential vitamins or minerals as such deficiencies will manifest themselves as problems in the future, such as anaemia from iron deficiency or osteoporosis (brittle bones) due to a lack of calcium.

Research, again carried out in Cambridge, showed that the following foods created symptoms of intolerance in the following percentages of patients:

- wheat, 60 per cent
- corn, 44 per cent
- milk, 44 per cent
- cheese, 39 per cent
- oats, 34 per cent
- coffee, 33 per cent
- rye, 30 per cent
- eggs, 26 per cent
- butter, 25 per cent
- tea, 25 per cent
- citrus, 24 per cent
- barley, 24 per cent
- yogurt, 24 per cent
- chocolate, 22 per cent
- nuts, 22 per cent
- onions, 22 per cent
- potatoes, 20 per cent
- preservatives, 20 per cent.

Probiotics and IBS

Researchers in Sweden have discovered that altering the gut flora by introducing probiotics ('good' bacteria) can significantly decrease the amount of pain and flatulence suffered in patients with IBS. To date the study of the influence of gut flora in people with IBS has not received much attention. The Swedish scientists recognized, however, that because some bacterial strains are more prone to gas production than others, if these can be reduced some relief of symptoms may be possible.

To test their theory, patients were given a fruit juice to drink which had been fortified with a member of the *Lactobacillus* family, a group of bacteria which are normally found in the healthy colon. By the end of the experiments, the scientists had been proven right. Adding *Lactobacillus plantarum* to the IBS sufferer's diet via the fruit juice had the effect of knocking out many of the gas-producing bacteria.

Flatulence decreased by half in 44 per cent of the group who had the drink with added probiotics. They also reported improved bowel movements. The drink is available in the UK under the name Proviva and can be found in good supermarkets.

'Alternative Testing'

It is possible to have a wide range of tests done that claim to prove food intolerances for IBS and other problems. Vega machines, hair analysis, cytotoxic tests – the list goes on. None has any scientific justification. Immunological abnormalities occur in some patients with known food intolerances. These can be detected by means of special tests, but they are notoriously tricky to do and can be unreliable.

Some scientists believe that food intolerances can develop due to a change in the flora in bowels due to antibiotic treatment in the past. Changes in flora have indeed been found in IBS patients who identify an aggravating food, remove it from the diet and then reintroduce it. Testing stools for changes in flora to detect food intolerances is not yet a recognized technique and it remains to be seen whether it could become so in the future.

The only reliable dietary treatment method available at the moment is that of following a proper exclusion diet under medical and dietetic supervision, such as the one suggested above.

Bloating

Bloating may be due to a food intolerance. Common intolerances that lead to bloating include an inability to deal with the milk sugar, lactose (for further details, see page 55).

Bloating can, however, be explained as being an occasional reaction to a certain type of food, such as cabbage or swede, or the result of an excessive amount of wind accumulating in the intestine. A sudden influx of high-fibre foods, especially pulses, can have this effect, too, while swallowing too much air is another cause. This last explanation may sound rather strange, but we all swallow air every time we speak, eat and drink. Eating in a rush, having large quantities of foods containing air, such as soufflés and meringues, and gulping down lots of carbonated drinks, all these things encourage extra air to be swallowed. However, this is easily remedied.

Dietary Advice

Again, the way in which you approach eating and drinking affects your digestion. Taking time and sitting down are essential. Chewing thoroughly and taking the whole process slowly will help reduce the amount of air swallowed with food. Gulping down foods and drinks will mean that you are taking in quite large quantities of air with each mouthful. Talking while eating has a similar effect, as does eating with your mouth open.

Avoid carbonated drinks. These introduce more unwanted air. Use plain water and still juices rather than fizzy water and orange, lemon, cola and other such drinks. It helps, too, to drink from a glass rather than straight from a bottle or can.

Chewing gum also causes you to swallow extra air. If you are having problems with excess wind, then try avoiding gum for a while to see if things improve at all.

When increasing the fibre content of your diet, remember to do so gradually. Start by making small, single changes, for example, just swapping from white to wholemeal bread. Gradually progress to including extra fruit and vegetables and, finally, start increasing the amounts of pulses, like beans and peas, in your diet. This allows the intestine time to get used to these foods and to produce the correct bacteria in the large intestine to deal with them, which will help keep the problem of bloating – which often accompanies a switch to a high-fibre diet – under control.

If bloating is a symptom of irritable bowel syndrome (IBS), see the previous section.

Candida

Candida albicans is one of the yeasts that we all have growing and living in our gut, and in women it is also found in the vagina. While most problems with overgrowth of *Candida* occur in the vagina, where it causes thrush, it can also affect the urinary tract and bladder, the throat, where it causes soreness, the mouth, leading to yellow patches and, when the immune system is under a lot of pressure, can affect other organs such as the eyes and liver. It also seems to affect the digestive system, causing bloating, pains and cramps, diarrhoea or IBS.

While *Candida* lives naturally in the gut, the strange thing is that those with a *Candida* problem don't appear to have any more of this yeast than those who don't suffer any adverse symptoms.

Possibly they just become more sensitive to normal levels. The important thing to note is that, whatever the reason, once patients try a low-sugar, low-yeast diet, symptoms of thrush often seem to disappear along with the intestinal symptoms of diarrhoea and wind. Your doctor can refer you to a dietitian who will advise you how to follow an appropriate diet.

Some trials have been carried out, with interesting results. One experiment, for example, showed that *Candida albicans* fails to grow in human saliva unless it is supplemented with glucose.

A trial was carried out in 1984 in which 100 women who had recurring *Candida* infections of the vagina had the sugar in their urine measured. When sugar appeared in the urine, it related to a time of excessive sugar intake. When sugar was eliminated as much as possible, there was a dramatic reduction in the incidence and severity of the *Candida* infections.

In an experimental study back in 1966, of 255 patients with long-term urticaria, 49 of them reacted to *Candida albicans* antigens, and 55 per cent of them also reacted to brewer's yeast. After treatment with a low-yeast diet and anti-fungal therapy, 27 out of the 49 experienced a clinical cure.

It has been suggested that a diet which excludes simple carbohydrate and yeast-rich foods will prevent candidiasis by depriving the organisms of a suitable environment in which to grow. This kind of diet requires the person involved to avoid foods containing simple sugars, which means no adding of sugar to foods or drinks at the table or eating foods rich in it, such as sweets, cakes, ice-creams and desserts, fruit juices, condiments and tinned fruits in syrup. It also involves cutting out yeast-containing foods and drinks, such as malted products, mushrooms, cheeses, peanuts and alcoholic drinks, as well as vinegar-containing foods and vitamin and mineral tablets, unless they are sugar- and yeast-free, and antibiotics.

The debate continues, but there are some respected clinics in which doctors and dietitians working together have seen improvements in patients who follow such diets and take the drug nystatin (prescribed for fungal infections).

Piles

Piles are largely believed to be related to over straining when trying to go to the loo. The best advice is to try to follow a high fibre diet and take plenty of fluids. See Constipation, page 68.

— 7 —

Cleansing the System of Poisons

Every day the digestive system is presented with 'foreign substances', such as bacteria and natural and chemical toxins, and it generally deals with these effectively and safely, killing them off, detoxifying them or simply coping with their presence. Sometimes, however, a food or drink may contain too much of a particular infectious or toxic agent, or be harbouring one against which the body has no defences.

When things get out of balance and poisoning occurs, the digestive tract plays an important role in eliminating the poison, by ejecting it from the system as quickly as possible. It does this by expelling the food from either the top or bottom of the tract by vomiting or diarrhoea. Less drastic symptoms of food poisoning include milder forms of indigestion, such as irritation of the mucous membranes, causing discomfort in the throat and/or the stomach, and feelings of nausea.

There are plenty of natural toxins in food that, in small amounts, we deal with effectively without suffering adverse effects. Ingesting them in large amounts, however, is a different matter. Solanine – the substance in green potatoes – is one such example.

Potatoes normally contain about 7 mg of solanine per 100-g (4-oz) serving. It is found mostly in green skin, but also in the eyes and sprouts of potatoes. It isn't enough just to cut off the green bits and remove the eyes, as the solanine can spread throughout the potato. When very small amounts of solanine are eaten, mild forms of poisoning occur that manifest themselves as general gastrointestinal discomfort, such as stomach ache and aches in the intestines, too. As the levels of solanine consumed rise, symptoms of nausea, vomiting and diarrhoea quickly set in. If levels of 33 mg per 100 g are reached, trouble really starts as the nervous system then becomes affected, with fever and the risk of circulatory collapse.

It is best to avoid potatoes with any sign of greening or sprouting. Always store them in a cool, dry, dark place to reduce the risk of solanine being produced, which happens when they are exposed to light for more than just a few days.

Toxins in poisonous mushrooms are another cause of vomiting and diarrhoea. *Amanita phalloides* is the mushroom most commonly responsible for poisoning in Britain. If only small amounts are ingested, you may get away with just abdominal pain.

Problems with mussels infected with saxitoxin are more likely than finding a rogue mushroom in your food, as there is no way of telling whether or not the mussel on your plate has fed on plankton containing the saxitoxin. Mussels themselves are not affected by it and, as it is not killed by cooking, it is only after eating a 'bad' one that you know because then you will be suffering from severe vomiting and diarrhoea.

As well as naturally occurring toxins, normally healthy foods and drinks can become infected by bacteria, which, once eaten, affect the digestive tract. Bacteria such as salmonella infect the intestines directly, causing upsets and aches, whereas others produce toxins and it is these toxins that do the damage, such as clostridium. The symptoms may be very severe and obviously linked to something recently consumed. Equally likely, however, are much milder levels of infection and these lead to general discomfort in the stomach and gut, feelings of nausea, queasiness and general indigestion, which won't be attributed to food poisoning.

Problems with food poisoning have always existed. The processing food undergoes now in the West attempts to reduce the risk by using a variety of techniques, such as pasteurization, canning and cooking, which all act as safeguards. The storage and handling of food and drink by the industry, retailer and ourselves at home play vital roles in keeping food poisoning under control.

Common Forms of Food Poisoning

Bacterial

Salmonella

Salmonella is the name given to a group of bacteria, of which there are more than 1,600 types. They are among the most common causes of food poisoning, infecting poultry and many other intensively reared animals. When we eat the infected meat, the bacteria are taken in with the food and usually stay in the intestinal tract where they wreak their havoc, causing pain, diarrhoea and vomiting. This usually begins around 12 to 36 hours after having eaten the contaminated food. It is quite common to be able to trace the symptoms back to a certain meal by checking how the people you ate with are feeling, as it is likely that all the people who ate the same food will be similarly affected. The digestive problems will usually last for up to two to three days.

Most cases of salmonella occur as a result of uncooked or badly cooked foods, or food that has been cooked and recontaminated. If, for example, an egg custard pie is cut with a knife that has been used for raw poultry and not thoroughly washed before being used again, the egg custard could easily become infected.

People can become carriers of salmonella. They have salmonella but don't have any symptoms, yet can pass the bacteria on to infect and affect others.

Basic Rules for Avoiding Salmonella Contamination

Meat and meat products, poultry, eggs, milk and milk products are the foods most commonly susceptible to salmonella contamination. If they are stored, handled and prepared properly, they do not pose a risk.

- When storing uncooked poultry, it should be kept in a fridge at less than 5°C and in a container that will not allow juices to drip on to foods below.
- Food should always be prepared with clean equipment and this should be thoroughly washed afterwards.
- Food should be cooked for long enough and at the correct temperatures.
- Cracked or damaged eggs should not be used and neither should those past the sell-by date. Dirty eggs should be wiped with a dry, clean cloth, but not washed as this destroys the protective film.
- Unpasteurized milk should be avoided.

Campylobacter

Stomach pains and discomfort followed by diarrhoea and fever are common symptoms of infection with campylobacter. The main type to infect the digestive system is *Campylobacter jejuni*. They are present in foods such as raw milk, some raw meats and poultry and unchlorinated water supplies. Campylobacter do not multiply in food, but once they enter the stomach and gut, they feed on what is for them a nutritionally rich medium that has the requisite low oxygen content and multiply with great speed. The symptoms are seldom serious and it is possible that an unexplained bout of indigestion could be down to mild infections with this bacteria.

The best way to avoid such infection is to consume only pasteurized or UHT milk, only drink water from known sources and avoid cross-contamination between cooked and uncooked foods. Heating does kill the bacteria, so cooked foods eaten hot are usually no problem.

Escherichia Coli

Consuming food or drink infected with *Escherichia coli* (usually simply *E. coli*) will again adversely affect the digestive tract. When the bacteria are ingested, they sit in the intestines and produce toxins, which lead to stomach pains, diarrhoea and maybe vomiting, too. The illness can last from one to seven days. Mild forms may cause cramps and indigestion that does not lead on to severe symptoms.

E. coli live in the large intestine and are transferred to food by means of poor personal hygiene. Simply thoroughly washing hands after going to the toilet and drying them on a clean towel is the best way of stopping them spreading. Meat can be infected with *E. coli* from humans or other animals. Care in handling is therefore vital to prevent infection.

Staphylococcus Aureus

Digestive tract symptoms of infection with *S. aureus* are similar to other types of food poisoning, including stomach cramps, nausea, diarrhoea and vomiting. The uppermost part of the digestive tract can also be affected, with excess saliva being produced. The bacteria produce a toxin that takes effect one to four hours after eating and can last for up to two days. *S. aureus* are found in the nasal passages of humans and animals and also often found in infected wounds and boils. They can also be passed from infected cattle into their milk.

As with *E. coli*, good hygiene can help avoid infections. Keeping hands clean and covering cuts and wounds is essential. Once the toxins have been produced, they cannot be destroyed by heating so preventing them from contaminating the food in the first place is vital. Poultry, meat, fish, milk and milk products are most susceptible to contamination with this bacteria.

Bacillus Cereus

If you become infected with *Bacillus cereus,* you will know about it all too soon. Usually within an hour, the bacteria have produced a toxin that will bring about waves of nausea and general discomfort in the stomach. If the poisoning is bad, sickness will follow within an hour and diarrhoea will start after eight hours.

B. cereus is found in the soil, but can find its way into the food chain. Once in food, the bacteria produce a toxin that actually only does the damage when the food is eaten. Boiled and fried rice are foods commonly affected by this bacteria, especially if cooked in bulk and left to stand for some time at normal room temperature. Custards, cereal products, puddings and sauces can also be affected.

The best way to avoid infection with *B. cereus* is to chill foods as quickly as possible once they have been cooked. Large quantities should be divided up into smaller amounts to speed up cooling and then be stored in the fridge. If reheated, it should be to temperatures above 70°c.

Moulds

Moulds are part of the fungi group of organisms. Most moulds are white and look furry or fuzzy, like fine cotton wool, although some are dark or coloured. Eating mouldy foods can upset the stomach and lead to vomiting and sickness.

Moulds usually turn foods bad and some also produce myco-toxins, which will cause harm when eaten. Some, however, are used in the food industry to make, for example, soy sauce and blue cheeses.

Mouldy foods should be thrown away. Scraping it off does not remove any toxins that may have been produced and have entered the food. Moulds are spread in the air as tiny spores that land on a food and multiply rapidly, which is another good reason for not disturbing it by cutting, but simply throw the whole piece away.

8

Cleansing and Calming the Gut Naturally

Self-cleansing of the gut does not require you to book an appointment for colonic irrigation. Manually evacuating the bowel disturbs the natural balance of bacteria which have built themselves up in the large intestine, and is generally regarded at best with scepticism by gastroenterologists, and at worst as a harmful practice.

This chapter on self-cleansing and calming is about learning how to take control of your digestive system and being kind to it. You can do this through ensuring your regular diet is well suited to your own particular digestive make-up, and by employing the use of herbs, supplements and foods with added ingredients designed specifically to improve intestinal health. It is also about taking time out to relax, de-stress and get yourself into good emotional shape.

The need to cleanse and calm the digestive system is nothing new. Since we first started roaming the planet, humans have been seeking the means by which to maintain and restore balance to their sensitive intestines. If you put together, in any combination, the potent forces of food, drink, overindulgence, intolerances, stress and anxiety, it's easy enough to work out why. Since digestive complaints are nothing new, it's not surprising that herbal medicine, which has been practised since time immemorial, has many remedies at its fingertips.

In addition to herbal solutions, basic good nutrition has a vital role to play in the repair and maintenance of the system. Some modern medical approaches to digestive problems also have their place.

Before trying any self-help or over-the-counter medications, check out your symptoms with your doctor to ensure your problems do not need medical or surgical intervention.

Cleansing

Water

Crucial to a healthy, cleansed gut is an adequate daily intake of water. You need it to digest food, dissolve nutrients so that they can pass through the intestinal cell walls into your bloodstream, and move food through the intestinal tract. Inadequate water can lead to constipation, especially when combined with a high-fibre diet. When the large intestine slows down its slow rhythmic movements, the bowel contents have the chance to stay in contact with the bowel wall for greater lengths of time, allowing potential toxins and cancer-causing substances to take a foothold. Looser, faster-moving, well-hydrated stools decrease the chances of this happening and thus reduce the risk of subsequent diseases whether they are infectious toxins or carcinogenic in origin.

Since the body does not have the ability to store water, a new supply must be taken daily, and this must be enough to replace losses from breath and perspiration (850–1,200 ml/30–42 fl oz), urination (600–1,600 ml/21–56 fl oz) and that lost through the stools (50 – 200 ml/2–7 fl oz): a grand total of 1½ —3 litres (3–6 US pints) of water a day.

Some of this water we get through food, but it is wise to try to drink around 2–2½ litres (4–5 US pints) a day. Bear in mind that not all liquids are equally liquefying. The caffeine in tea and coffee and the alcohol in alcoholic drinks have a diuretic effect, which makes you urinate more and thus lose some of the benefits of the liquid part of the drink.

People who eat a lot of salt and those taking exercise need to increase fluid intakes. After an hour's exercise you can lose a good litre (35 fl oz) of body water through perspiration. It is important to keep drinking throughout the day. Remember, by the time your mouth is dry and you are registering thirst, you are already dehydrated.

If you become dehydrated through lack of access to fluids or perhaps through diarrhoea, the quickest way to rehydrate is with isotonic sports drinks such as Lucozade Sport or Gatorade. You can make your own version by taking a glass of squash or concentrated fruit juice and adding a pinch of salt.

Probiotics

Altering the balance of undesirable bacteria in favour of the health-enhancing varieties is a concept with which we are becoming familiar. This cleansing of the large intestine from the inside out is a growing market with more and more products, most of which are milk- and dairy-based, on supermarket shelves. 'Live yogurts' have made their way out of the specialist health food stores and now sit proudly alongside established brands. We even see little Japanese fermented milk available by the tills of the local shop.

The key to an effective probiotic is knowing that the bacteria can survive the acidic stomach environment, the alkaline conditions of the duodenum, and be able to make it to the large intestine. Few in practice are able to do this. Once in the bowel, the probiotic needs to be able to attach itself to the wall and successfully reproduce.

Intensive research carried out in Sweden has shown that five of the 20 or so different strains of *Lactobacilli* bacteria which are commonly present in the intestine have this ability. Scientists have proved that of these five, *Lactobacillus plantarum* 299v adheres particularly well to the intestinal wall and reduces the number of anaerobic bacteria and toxin-producing clostridia which are particularly problematic in the gut. *Lactobacillus plantarum* 299v helps to cleanse and rebalance the gut after courses of antibiotics, chronic diarrhoea, inflammatory intestinal diseases, cramps and post-operative infections. It can also be taken on a daily basis as a protective measure. This unique and effective probiotic is available in a fruit juice-based drink known as Proviva. Being non-dairy, it is the first effective probiotic available to those who are milk-intolerant.

Soluble and Insoluble Fibre

There cannot be a more natural way of spring cleaning your digestive tract than increasing your intake of fibrous foods. Starting in the mouth, foods rich in fibre give the teeth and gums a physical workout. Once in the stomach, both soluble fibrous fractions (found in oats, beans, apples and pears) and insoluble fractions (in wholegrain cereals and some vegetables) can wrap up potential disease-forming substances and sweep them out of the system.

Certain soluble fibres which form gels in the small intestine can bind bacteria to them so that both leave the gut via the stools. Insoluble fibres, on the other hand, literally absorb potentially harmful cancer-inducing substances. They do so by binding water to their surface and trapping the baddies within the bulky stools. Fibre is also capable of diluting carcinogens lurking within the colonic contents and moving them swiftly out of the gut.

Nourishing the Tract Itself

Since the digestive tract is surrounded for its entire length by muscles, not surprisingly nutrients which feed and nurture muscular tissue are important to the system's ability to keep moving at the correct pace. Equally, vitamins and minerals that are essential for the correct functioning of the nerves and hormones which regulate muscle movement must be supplied in adequate amounts if the system is to keep moving.

A diet rich in carbohydrates, as found in bread, cereals, rice, pasta, potatoes and fruits, provides muscles with a constant source of energy in the form of glucose and the stored form of glucose, glycogen. Dairy products, nuts, seeds, dark green vegetables and dried fruits supply both calcium and magnesium, minerals needed by muscle fibres to contract and relax, thus creating the peristaltic waves which move the digested food contents along.

For the nervous system, a good and constant supply of B vitamins are needed, especially B_6 (in meat, milk and potatoes) and B_{12} (in meat, dairy products, fish, eggs and fortified soya milks and breakfast cereals). Folic acid is also important, and can be found in wholegrain cereals, fortified breads and cereals and Marmite (yeast extract).

Herbal Cleansers

Herbs can provide a simple yet effective way of cleansing various parts of the digestive system.

The Mouth

For cleansing the mouth, try adding 5 ml (about 1 teaspoonful) of myrrh tincture to a glass of warm water and use as a mouthwash to benefit from its antimicrobial properties. A similar quantity of bistort tincture can be added to water for an astringent cleanse, or try 10 ml of sage tincture diluted in water – this has antiseptic qualities and is thus good for helping fight gum disorders and gingivitis.

The Large Intestine

To lubricate and bulk the bowel contents to help flush them through, try infusing a teaspoon of psyllium seeds or linseeds in a cup of boiling water. Allow them to cool and drink with the seeds twice daily. To speed gut contents, take 2 ml of rhubarb tincture three times a day. The antraquinones in the rhubarb irritate the gut lining and increase its movements.

Sorbitol is a sugar alcohol found in some fruits, such as plums, apricots, cherries and apples. It is made for commercial use from fruit sugars and is added to many sugar-free products. Sorbitol is absorbed quite slowly from the intestine and tends to draw water into it. If eaten in large amounts – a tube of sugar-free mints in one sitting, for example – it can stimulate bowel contractions and lead to a fast clear-out of the colon contents.

The same is true of prunes, which contain derivatives of a substance called hydroxyphenylizaton that directly stimulates the smooth muscle of the colon wall.

Other foods which have this natural laxative effect include rhubarb, figs, liquorice, molasses, senna and castor oil.

Nurturing

The Gut Lining

Keeping the lining of the digestion system in good condition from the mouth right down to the rectum and anus is important for many reasons, from helping to prevent mouth ulcers to stopping the colon becoming 'leaky' and thus allowing dangerous bacteria to move from the tract into the blood and set up life-threatening infections in other organs.

Vitamin A, as found in liver (not suitable for pregnant women), whole dairy products, eggs, carrots and dark green vegetables, and vitamin E as found in wheatgerm, avocados and nuts, are both needed for membrane health. So too are the essential fatty acids (EFAs) found in oily fish, flax seed oil and evening primrose oil.

To soothe an irritated stomach lining you need to avoid foods and drinks which increase stomach acid secretion. These include alcohol, caffeine and hot spicy foods. Try a tincture of meadowsweet or liquorice, both of which are anti-inflammatory. The former soothes and heals the stomach lining while the latter helps to produce a viscous mucus which coats the stomach wall and reduces acid secretion.

An inflamed lining can also be helped by the essential fatty acids in fish and evening primrose oil, which both act by suppressing the pro-inflammatory substances.

For the large intestine, regularly taking probiotics (see page 93) strengthens the gut wall bacteria and allows them to fight off potentially dangerous invaders.

Enzyme Release

For the intestine to carry out its primary function of digesting and absorbing foods, the enzymes which do the physical breaking down need to be in plentiful supply and their secretion under proper control. Zinc from red meats and wholegrain foods, magnesium from milk products, selenium from brazil nuts, cereals and fish, and copper from wholemeal bread and vegetables are all important for the activation of these enzymes.

Calming

The tremendous effects (both perceptible and imperceptible) which the nerves surrounding the intestines and those in the central nervous system have on the physical functioning of the digestive tract should never be underestimated. When you have been through or find yourself experiencing a stressful period in your life, then you can be sure that your gut will feel the effects. To calm things down there is much that can be done, both by turning to the world of herbs and looking at alternative forms of exercise and meditation.

Herbal Helpers

For general anxiety and tension an infusion, tincture or capsules of skullcap are often recommended by herbalists. Infusions or tinctures of linden or vervain may also prove useful. To aid relaxation, tinctures of mugwort, gotu kola, lavender or camomile can be taken. Lemon balm tea and valerian tablets offer another option.

Alternative Therapies for Calming the Nervous System

Acupuncture

Originating in China, acupuncture is based on the concept that disease involves an imbalance within the body systems. Treatment is intended to restore equilibrium and balance; it is achieved by inserting appropriate needles in exactly the right places (along points known as meridians) by the practitioners. The nervous system is said to respond well to this form of treatment. Usually within seconds of the needles being positioned, a deeply relaxed – even drowsy – state is experienced. For the most part acupuncture in the UK is not available on the NHS and you will need to find a qualified, private practitioner should you wish to try this therapy.

Aromatherapy

This makes use of a combination of body and face massage using essential oils extracted from plants. It can be practised as an extension of herbalism or simply as part of a beauty massage. In aromatherapy it is the aromatic oils which give plants their distinctive smells (the essences) that are used. These can come from the roots, flowers, leaves, bark or resin, and no two are alike. In the plants themselves these essences serve particular functions such as acting as pesticides, fungicides and bactericides, and are often used in the cosmetics and toiletries we use daily. Aroma-therapists use these essences, massaging them into the skin. These essences then make their way into the body's extra-cellular fluids.

Oils of melissa and rosemary have a calming effect when used in a specific dose. For nervous tension, bergamot, camphor, camomile, rose, ylang-ylang, sandalwood and orange blossom are among the first choices. A massage with these oils will prove relaxing and also help calm inner tensions and stress.

Biofeedback Training

This treatment involves training the body to modify specific activities with the benefit of experience. A biofeedback expert can train you to increase particular types of brain waves to make you feel relaxed and pleasant. Biofeedback opens up tremendous scope to us as individuals to control our reactions and moods, especially when we know we are going to be plunged into a stressful situation.

Hypnosis

Hypnosis alters the state of the mind but does *not* send you to sleep. A session of hypnotherapy can leave you deeply relaxed. Direct suggestion therapy is a good place to start.

Massage

Massage in all its forms can have the most tremendously comforting, de-stressing effects on the body. Feeling cosseted, cared for and soothed helps even the most uptight person relax, and leaves a person feeling calm, refreshed and revitalized.

There are many different types of massage techniques, one of which is bound to suit you as an individual. You could, for example, try Reiki, for which the practitioner has been attuned to act as a channel for 'Ki', meaning 'life-force'. Ki is drawn from the masseur's hands to exactly where the recipient needs it, helping to clean the body of toxins and create a state of balance on the physical, emotional and spiritual levels.

Shiatsu is another option. Literally meaning 'finger pressure', it is a form of Japanese massage and pressure designed to stimulate the acupuncture points and meridians. In some ways we all already know about the practice of shiatsu. When a mother rubs a child's bruised leg better or we soothe our own knocks and bumps by rubbing the injured site with our hands, it is the transference of healing powers at work, and this is what shiatsu is all about. A good practitioner can use the technique to calm even the most strung-out individuals.

Yoga

The word yoga means 'oneness' in Sanskrit; it is a personal self-help system for both physical and spiritual health. Learning the postures and breathing techniques can help us unravel many ailments and the emotional knots we tie ourselves up in. With practice it is possible to alter your heart rate and blood pressure and find a wonderful sense of relaxation. Specific postures can actually help to improve ailments of the digestive tract.

Orthodox Remedies for Disturbed Digestion

For the Stomach

Until recently, neutralization of the acidic conditions in the stomach had been the only way to deal with indigestion in this part of the tract, and this method has been used for several centuries. More recently it has been discovered that it is possible to control the actual production of acid in a very specific way. It is also recognized that in addition to controlling the production of acid, it is worth looking into ways of fortifying the usual protective mechanism of the stomach – the mucous membranes.

Controlling the acidity in the stomach is an important part of the treatment for ulcers and severe acid reflux.

Neutralizing Acids – Antacids

Antacid literally means anti-acid, and antacid medicines are designed to neutralize the acid in the stomach. The various ones are therefore made from one or more alkaline substances. Liquid preparations work fastest, but tablets are more convenient to carry around.

By neutralizing the acid in the stomach, antacids produce two desirable effects. They decrease the total amount of acid that moves on into the duodenum and stop the activity of pepsin (one of the enzymes in the stomach juices that breaks down protein). Over long periods, all antacids can have side-effects, so they shouldn't be taken for more than two weeks or so. With those you can buy over the counter at your pharmacist, it is best to check with your doctor before taking them and essential to do so if you are pregnant or breastfeeding, on a low-sodium diet, suffer from heart, blood pressure, liver or kidney problems, or take other medicines on a regular basis.

There are two main types of antacids. Those which are absorbed into the bloodstream and are therefore capable of increasing the pH level of the blood as well as the stomach, which leads to alkaline urine being produced. Then there are the ones that are not absorbed and so do not affect the blood. These are preferable to the absorbed kind if the medicine is to be taken over a couple of weeks.

What is in antacids?

- *Baking soda* Known chemically as sodium bicarbonate or sodium carbonate, these are fast and effective antacids, although they can wear off quickly. They can also lead to belching because they produce carbon dioxide in the stomach. The sodium content makes them out of bounds for anyone with a heart condition, high blood pressure, liver or kidney problems. These antacids are the type that are absorbed into the bloodstream.

- *Chalk* The chemical name for chalk is calcium carbonate. Like baking soda, chalk is an effective antacid. It does release carbon dioxide as it sets to work, however, and can lead to constipation, so it should not be taken for long periods. It is capable of interacting with other medicines like antibiotics, too, so, again, check with your doctor before taking. These antacids are not absorbed into the bloodstream.

- *Aluminium hydroxide* This is less effective than the two above. Like chalk, it has a constipating effect, so it is usually available in a preparation that also contains magnesium, which has a laxative effect so they cancel each other out. This type of antacid must be avoided if you have kidney problems and is known to interact with some antibiotics, antifungal drugs, warfarin and digoxin.

- *Magnesium carbonate, magnesium trisilicate, magnesium hydroxide* These are effective antacids, but they have a laxative effect. They are usually found in combination with calcium or aluminium and are another type that should be avoided if you have kidney problems.

These are the main active ingredients in antacids, but they also contain other ingredients to help relieve various symptoms.

- *Dimethicone or simethicone* This is added to help break up the gas bubbles, although there is little really good evidence regarding its effectiveness. It is supposed to work by allowing the gas bubbles to coalesce (join together) and then be expelled.
- *Alginic acid* This comes from seaweed and, when it reaches the stomach, forms into a foamy gel. This gel works by sitting as a raft on top of the stomach's contents, preventing them from refluxing out of the stomach and back up into the oesophagus.

Antacids are useful for helping ulcers to heal, if taken properly. Their disadvantage is that they have to be taken regularly and, as mentioned, have side-effects. The chalky taste most of them have is often poorly accepted, which means that people tend to stop taking them before they have had their beneficial effect and healing has been completed. It would seem that antacids are not as safe as some of the newer treatments, which actually stop the acid being produced in the first place.

Blocking Acid Production

How acid is produced and secreted into the stomach was described earlier, but, to refresh our memories, it is controlled by several mechanisms.

1. Nerve stimulation, which can be triggered by the sight, smell and taste of food and its arrival in the stomach. The particular nerve involved is the vagus nerve, which releases a substance called acetycholine and this fixes on to a special receptor site in the acid-secreting parietal cells in the stomach wall. This action then stimulates acid secretion.

2. By a hormone called gastrin. Gastrin is released from the mucous membranes of the stomach when food is present. The gastrin latches on to its own special gastrin receptor sites in the parietal cell to stimulate acid secretion.

3. By the action of a substance called histamine, which itself is stimulated by the presence of food in the stomach and by acetylcholine and gastrin. Histamine latches on to a histamine receptor in the acid-secreting parietal gland.

When just one of these three stimulators fixes on to the parietal cell, the secretion of acid is scanty. When all three fix on to it, though, the acid literally pours into the stomach.

Mechanisms to reduce acid secretion therefore involve blocking the substances that cause the parietal cells to release it. These are the following.

Anticholinergics

These drugs stop the impulses from the vagus nerve getting to the acid-secreting cells in the stomach wall. They are able to reduce acid secretion but do not stop it completely.

Anticholinergics were known to have various side-effects. For example, some people found they developed blurred vision, others developed a dry mouth, making chewing and swallowing difficult. Small doses may still be used, but, in the main, they have been replaced by the following more modern treatments.

H$_2$ Antagonists

These substances are able to latch on to the histamine receptor site on the parietal cell and effectively prevent the histamine latching on. If no histamine is locked on to the receptor, the parietal cell will not release any acid. It's rather like blocking someone's keyhole up with filler or glue – there is then no way for them to get their key into the door and thus turn it to enter. H$_2$ receptor blockers, or antagonists, as they are called, include substances with names like famotidine, cimetidine and ranitidine and block all three stimulators of the acid-secreting cell.

H$_2$ blockers work by reducing the background level of acid during the day and night in the stomach, as well as the amount of acid that is released during the day in response to eating and drinking, and even just thinking about food. The decrease in acid secretion that results from this blocking allows the mucous membranes, in particular the duodenal ones, to tolerate the lower acidity of the material it receives from the stomach, which gives the ulcer a better chance of healing, improves the speed at which healing occurs and helps prevent the recurrence of ulcers.

Side-effects of these medicines are usually rare and minor, although people with kidney problems do need to take them in lower doses. There can also be interaction with other medication, like warfarin, so, again, care needs to be taken.

The H$_2$ receptor sites are not the same as the histamine receptor sites in the airways and air passages – these are H$_1$ sites. These are not therefore affected by the H$_2$ antagonist drugs used to treat indigestion.

Proton Pump Inhibitors

Once the sites on the parietal cell have been locked on to, whether it is by acetylcholine, gastrin or histamine, all then go on to cause hydrochloric acid to be secreted into the stomach by a pump action. There is a group of drugs that can interfere with this final part of the process so that even if the receptor sites have been stimulated, acid production can still be stopped. These drugs are called proton pump inhibitors.

They produce a more rapid response and promote a faster rate of healing of ulcers than H_2 antagonists and are particularly good for people suffering from refluxing up into the throat or oesophagus. They can, however, cause side-effects, including headaches, rashes and diarrhoea.

Antibiotics

Since the emergence of the theory that stomach ulcers may be caused by the bacteria *Helicobacter pylori* (*H. pylori*), many doctors now treat stomach and duodenal ulcers with a cocktail of drugs. Such a cocktail would include an antibiotic, taken for a week or two, to eradicate the bacteria, and an H_2 blocker, such as cimetidine, famotidine or ranitidine to control acid secretion and give the ulcerated region a chance to heal. Such treatment seems to work very effectively.

Mucus-protecting Agents

Another group of substances can help, too – the cytoprotectants. They act by increasing the secretion of the protective mucus and bicarbonate, and/or by actually providing a physical barrier, thus covering up the ulcer, preventing further irritation of the area to aid healing.

Sucralfate, for example, is thought to act by coating the ulcer, by forming a sticky substance which protects against acid, pepsin and bile salts. It also stimulates the production of mucus, bicarbonate and prostaglandins. It is effective in helping the healing of ulcers.

Another long name to remember is carbenoxolone sodium. This helps the healing of gastric and duodenal ulcers along by improving mucosal defence. It is not the usual first choice in ulcer treatment because of the availability of other more modern drugs that have effective track records. Carbenoxolone sodium is not suitable for children, pregnant women, the elderly or those with heart, kidney or liver problems.

Pharmacy Availability of H_2 Blockers

Doctors have been able to prescribe H_2 blockers for some years. Some well-known ones are Tagamet (cimetidine), Zantac (ranitidine) and Pepcid (famotidine). However, it is now possible to buy weaker versions from the chemists as an 'over-the-counter' product – in other words, you ask the pharmacist for it. The pharmacist should run through a checklist before allowing you to have it, though, to check that it is safe for you to take.

9

You're Not Alone

If you suffer with digestive problems then you most definitely are not alone. In the UK alone around 14 million people at any one time are experiencing problems with bloating, aching, bouts of wind and general discomfort. These problems can disrupt pleasure and leisure time, work, sleep and the ability to enjoy food and drink.

One of the largest surveys carried out to discover more about such complaints questioned 1,004 people to gain an insight into causes and how people deal with their problems. Men and women, it was discovered, suffer in equal amounts and no age group remained untouched by symptoms, although people between the ages of 35 and 64 were the most affected. Those in professional occupations were most prone to attacks, followed by managerial and manual workers. Of all the people questioned, 80 per cent could relate their digestive problems to a particular cause.

Problem Foods

The foods listed here were those perceived to provoke negative digestive reactions.

- fatty foods, 58 per cent
- spicy foods, 47 per cent
- alcohol, 39 per cent
- fizzy drinks, 37 per cent
- rich foods, 31 per cent
- onions, 29 per cent
- peppers, 24 per cent
- citrus fruits, 23 per cent
- fruit juice, 20 per cent
- garlic, 17 per cent
- tomatoes, 13 per cent
- chocolate, 13 per cent
- coffee, 12 per cent
- food containing air, 9 per cent
- cabbage, 6 per cent.

Women seemed to be more aware of which particular types of foods triggered their indigestion than were men. Fatty foods, for example, were more frequently pinpointed by women than men. Spicy foods, second on the list, were, again, mentioned more often by women than men.

Alcohol and fizzy drinks came next. Alcohol was the second most common cause stated by men, and, in fact, the only factor mentioned significantly more often by men than women. The difficulties caused by alcohol follow the general trends seen in alcohol consumption. Men and those in work mentioned this cause more often than other groups. The older respondents had less trouble with alcohol sparking off indigestion, which is in line with the general drop in alcohol consumption in this group.

Rich foods were unspecified but acknowledged by a significant number of the people asked to be a contributing factor to their digestive upsets.

Among the individual foods mentioned, onions and peppers were the most frequently pinpointed. The survey revealed that indigestion following eating citrus fruit was more of a problem in older people and they mentioned fruit juices as a cause more often, too. Less frequently mentioned were problems triggered by garlic, tomatoes, chocolate and coffee. Those who thought eating foods with air in them were to blame named popcorn and meringues as potential causes.

The people taking part in the survey were then asked what they avoided because it gave them indigestion. The answers they gave are shown below in perceived order of importance.

Factor	Percentage who avoided it
Overeating/eating too quickly	85
Stress	59
Putting on weight	58
Eating before bed	58
Exercising after meals	55
Tight clothing	51
Eating fast foods	49
Smoking	31
Bending	30

Stress

Of the people taking part in the survey, almost 60 per cent said that stress played a big role in digestive upsets. Family problems lay at the heart of many of the cases. For women, juggling the commitments of children, elderly relatives, holding down a job and coping with family life were triggers. Adjusting lifestyles was one of the key factors they felt needed addressing. Take a look at some of the suggestions in Chapter 7 to help you take control and make changes to your current way of life.

Other Factors

Overeating and eating too rapidly were other key areas which people identified as being a source of their digestive turmoil. Wearing tight clothes, laying down after eating and pregnancy were also said to be triggers. Clearly these are all things which can be addressed by the individual. Making time for meals and snacks is crucial. Try planning ahead and giving yourself, at the very least, five minutes each side of eating. Keep your tight clothes for special occasions, and avoid wearing them when you know you will be expected to eat a large meal.

Self-Help

Keeping symptoms to ourselves seems to be one of the key features of digestive disorders. Most people seem to find ways of coping without making a fuss. Some turn to orthodox treatments and do not make any attempt to change eating habits or lifestyles, while others take positive steps to get to the root of the problem. It is crucial that before turning to the kind of solutions outlined in the case histories below, that you first consult with your doctor so that he or she can rule out any underlying problems which need to be dealt with through medical or surgical intervention.

Caroline, 32: Stress-related Stomach Cramps

A fashion buyer for a large chain store, Caroline works long hours at an unrelentingly fast pace. Her job demands a lot of travel and out-of-hours entertaining.

'I suppose my digestive system is uptight from the moment I open my eyes in the morning. I know the rushed feeling must get transferred to all my internal organs including my stomach. I don't have breakfast because the butterfly feeling stops me wanting to eat, and whenever I do have something, experience tells me I rush it down and feel uncomfortable for the rest of the morning. The same pretty much goes for lunch, a bolted sandwich seems to give me stomach cramps, pain and bloating, so unless I'm with clients it's usually just a piece of fruit which I grab on the go. Dinner is usually at a restaurant where most of the foods on offer are rich, and if I'm feeling nervous about the people I'm dining with because they are important to business then I know I'll pay for my meal with a bad stomach later.

'I can honestly say the only time I enjoy food is at the weekend when I can eat the foods I enjoy and do so at my own pace. I know that there is nothing seriously wrong with me, partly because my doctor told me so but more because I feel fine when I'm able to relax. I was advised by a friend to start taking yoga classes so that I could learn how to breathe in a controlled way which helps to lower your heart rate. It's not easy but I am gradually getting the hang of it. If I remember to take five minutes to calm down before a lunch I think my stomach seems to cope better. It's a bit like massaging out a taut muscle, I suppose. It's the only solution I can think of because I certainly don't want to change my job.'

Jenny, 35: Yeast and Sugar Intolerance-induced Bloating, Wind and Thrush

A television executive with a five-year history of thrush and digestive complaints, Jenny finally discovered she was intolerant to sugar and yeast. Diet was the key to her recovery.

'I kept getting bouts of thrush due to a problem with Candida. It was really getting me down and I was fed up with taking medicine which

didn't seem to knock it out. It was this which finally led my doctor to refer me to a dietitian, who helped me look at things with a fresh perspective. I was surprised at how draconian her advice was, but I decided that I had better give it a try. She literally made me stop eating all foods containing yeast, which included everything from bread and wine to less obvious things like grapes and plums, cheese, crumpets and even cream crackers. I also had to give up all sugar – and I mean all *sugar. I couldn't believe that here was a dietitian telling me not to eat fruit! The diet was difficult to follow and I lapsed a few times. However, my thrush really did start to go. Not only that, the dreadful bloating and wind which I had thought was just a part of everyday life also started to subside.*

'I am not as strict about sugar now but I still avoid eating too many yeast-containing foods. I can cope with the odd glass of wine and about two slices of toast a day. I know my limits and I really do stay within them.'

Elizabeth, 54: Irritable Bowel Following Hysterectomy

Elizabeth, an active and sociable housewife, had a hysterectomy when she was 52 and within weeks was suffering bowel symptoms she had never previously experienced.

'I was expecting to feel weak and under the weather for a while after my operation, but to my surprise it wasn't the actual hysterectomy which caused a lot of pain, rather the odd way my bowels started to behave. It was about six weeks after the surgery, during which time I was taking antibiotics for an infection. Quite out of the blue I noticed terrible swings between going to the loo far more often than normal and not going for days on end. The bloating was also bad, but I put this down to the operation.

'I was sent to see a specialist in Irritable Bowel Syndrome, who talked about it being related to emotional problems. I had to be quite tough with him and insisted I was not about to have a breakdown and that I was completely happy with my husband. We don't have any real worries, so eventually he ruled that out. I think he was just testing me out, because very soon after he turned to what I ate and asked me about my favourite foods. I eat a lot of dairy products and bread.

'It was the bread which struck a chord with him. He explained that sometimes the foods we like most can be responsible for changes in bowel habits. That this started after my hysterectomy apparently is not uncommon. It is something to do with the drugs I took and possibly the body's reaction to the whole process of being interfered with.

'Anyway, I've been avoiding wheat in bread but also have had to give up cakes and biscuits, some breakfast cereals and even pies and pasta. Everything is a lot better so it has been worth it, although at times I have felt really rude saying no all the time to the things I love eating when I'm at other people's houses or out to dinner in a nice restaurant.'

Tony, 29: Constant Problems with Heartburn

Tony's job as a taxi driver means he is sitting down virtually all day and gets very little exercise. He eats his lunch on the hoof, grabbing fast foods where and when he gets the chance. His weight has been increasing since he gave up sports and started cabbing.

'Some days I don't know how I kept going. I used to eat a constant supply of mints to keep that acidy feeling out of my throat, and chewed those antacid things like they were going out of fashion. It didn't get any better, though, and there were moments when the pain got so bad I thought I was having a heart attack. The doctor, like my wife, kept on at me to lose weight. He said that the weight, combined with sitting down all day, was the cause of the problem. I'm 17 stone (238 lb) and 5'10", so I'm on the hefty side for someone my age.

'In the end I joined weight watchers. I've heard all the jokes but it is working. I've learned about various foods I can eat plenty of, and various ones I need to be strict with. My wife gives me stuff to take with me and I've knocked the burgers and what-not on the head. Eventually she also persuaded me to see this friend of hers who's into herbs. I've got these little brown bottles of potions we keep in the fridge, and I even drink camomile tea. To be honest the acidy feeling is going. If you'd told me a few years ago that shifting some weight and taking a few herbs could help, I'd have laughed. I thought the old heartburn was my lot in life. Something I had to get used to. It wasn't. I'm beating it and I'm happy about that.'

— 10 —
The Recipes

All recipes are for one person, unless otherwise indicated.

Low-acid Recipes for Heartburn, Stomach Ulcers and Stomach Cramps

These recipes avoid the use of foods which cause extra acid secretions, such as certain spices and onions. They are designed to be kind on the stomach.

Breakfasts

Baked Banana with Fromage Frais and Toasted Muffin

1 large banana, peeled	1 large banana, peeled
1½ tsp dark brown sugar	1½ tsp dark brown sugar
1 tbsp mango juice	1 tbsp mango juice
2 tbsp low-fat fromage frais	1 tbsp low-fat fromage blanc
1 wholemeal muffin, sliced in half	1 wholewheat English muffin, sliced in half
2 tsp low-fat spread	2 tsp low-fat spread

Pre-heat the oven to 200°C/400°F/gas 6.

Take a rectangle of foil large enough to wrap the banana in loosely. Lay the banana on the foil, sprinkle with the sugar and mango juice, then scrunch up the foil around the banana and bake in the pre-heated oven for 10 minutes. Unwrap and serve in the foil with the fromage frais.

Follow the baked banana with the muffin, toasted, topped with the spread.

Grilled Mushrooms on Sunflower Seed Toast

4 flat mushrooms	4 flat mushrooms
2 thick slices wholegrain bread with sunflower seeds or wholemeal bread	2 thick slices wholegrain bread with sunflower seeds or wholewheat bread
2 tsp low-fat spread	2 tsp low-fat spread
salt and freshly ground black pepper	salt and freshly ground black pepper
pinch of celery salt	pinch of celery salt
200 ml (⅓ pint) carrot juice, chilled	scant cup carrot juice, chilled

Wipe the mushrooms clean and grill. Toast the bread, spread the low-fat spread over, arrange the mushrooms on the toast and season to taste.

Stir a pinch of celery salt into the carrot juice and serve.

Boiled Eggs with Bread

1 egg	1 egg
2 slices wholemeal bread	2 slices wholewheat bread
2 tsp low-fat spread	2 tsp low-fat spread
1 tsp marmalade	1 tsp marmalade
200 ml (⅓ pint) mango juice, chilled	scant cup mango juice, chilled
2–3 ice cubes	2–3 ice cubes

Boil the egg and serve with a slice of the wholemeal bread, spread with half of the low-fat spread.

Have the second slice of bread topped with the rest of the spread and the marmalade.

Crush the ice cubes in a tea towel with a wooden rolling pin (or just use whole) and place in a tall glass. Add the chilled mango juice and serve.

Blackberry Fruit Shake

100 g (4 oz) blackberries, fresh or frozen	scant cup blackberries, fresh or frozen
small pot of low-fat plain yogurt	small pot of low-fat plain yogurt
200 ml (⅓ pint) skimmed milk	scant cup skim milk
2 slices fruit loaf	2 slices raisin bread

Defrost the blackberries if using frozen. Blend together the blackberries, yogurt and skimmed milk. Serve chilled in a tall glass.

Either toast the fruit loaf slices or have them untoasted, as you prefer, and serve them with the shake.

Peach and Pear Yogurt and Wholemeal Toast

1 ripe peach	1 ripe peach
1 ripe pear	1 ripe pear
1 small pot (150 ml/¼ pint) plain low-fat yogurt	½ cup plain low-fat yogurt
1 tsp honey	1 tsp honey
slice of wholemeal toast	slice of wholewheat toast
butter	butter
marmalade	marmalade

Finely chop the peach and pear and mix together in a bowl. Pour over the yogurt, then and drizzle over a teaspoon of honey. Serve this fruit yogurt mix followed by the slice of toast with a little butter and marmalade. Have with a glass of mineral water.

Lunches

Chicken Roll with Lettuce

1 wholemeal roll	1 wholewheat roll
1 tsp low-fat spread	1 tsp low-fat spread
80 g (3 oz) cooked chicken	3 oz cooked chicken
freshly ground black pepper	freshly ground black pepper
2–3 lettuce leaves	2–3 lettuce leaves
3 rings red pepper	3 rings red bell pepper
1 tsp reduced-fat salad cream or mayonnaise	1 tsp reduced-fat salad cream or mayonnaise
1 medium peach	1 medium peach
60 g (2½ oz) ice-cream	2½ oz ice-cream

Split the roll and spread the low-fat spread on the lower half. Lay the cooked chicken on top. Grind over some black pepper, then add the lettuce and pepper rings. Spread the salad cream or mayonnaise on the other half of the roll and place on top of the filling.

For dessert, slice up the peach and serve with the ice-cream.

Watercress Soup with French Bread

2 bunches watercress	2 bunches watercress
a few fresh tarragon fronds	a few fresh tarragon fronds
550 ml (18 fl oz) water	2¼ cups water
salt and freshly ground black pepper	salt and freshly ground black pepper
115 ml (4 fl oz) skimmed milk	½ cup skim milk
120 g (4½ oz) chunk French bread	4½ oz chunk French bread
1 medium nectarine	1 medium nectarine

Put the watercress and fresh tarragon in a pan. Add the water, season to taste, bring to the boil and simmer very gently, covered, for 25 minutes.

Blend, then add the milk and simmer for 10 more minutes. Check the seasoning, allow to cool, then chill.

Serve a quarter of the soup with the French bread. Chill or freeze the rest of the soup.

Have the nectarine for dessert.

Turkey Club Sandwich

1 tsp low-fat spread	1 tsp low-fat spread
3 slices wholemeal bread	3 slices wholewheat bread
75 g (3 oz) cooked lean turkey	3 oz cooked lean turkey

1 tsp horseradish sauce or to taste	1 tsp horseradish sauce or to taste
1 tsp reduced-fat salad cream or mayonnaise	1 tsp reduced-fat salad cream or mayonnaise
1 lettuce leaf, washed	1 lettuce leaf, washed
4 slices cucumber	4 slices cucumber
1 apple	1 apple

Use the spread on one slice of bread. Place the roast beef on top and spread with the horseradish sauce to taste. Lay the second slice of bread on top of this. Spread the salad cream or mayonnaise on this piece of bread and lay the lettuce and slices of cucumber on top. Add the final piece of bread, hold firmly and cut diagonally into four. Put a cocktail stick through each quarter to stop the sections toppling over.

Have the apple for dessert.

Greek Salad with Hot Bread

40 g (1½ oz) feta cheese, cubed	1½ oz feta cheese, cubed
4 black olives, stoned	4 black olives, pitted
2 tomatoes, chopped	2 tomatoes, chopped
1 in (2.5 cm) chunk cucumber, diced	1 in chunk cucumber, diced
1 tbsp oil-free French dressing	1 tbsp oil-free French dressing
80 g (3 oz) chunk French bread	3 oz chunk French bread
1 small pear	1 small pear

Put the feta cheese into a bowl with the olives, tomatoes and cucumber. Pour the French dressing over and mix. Warm the bread and serve with the salad.

Have the pear for dessert.

Crunchy Camembert Baguette

100 g (4 oz) baguette	4oz baguette
40 g (1½ oz) Camembert	1½ oz Camembert
2 tsp cranberry sauce	2 tsp cranberry sauce
shredded iceberg lettuce	shredded iceberg lettuce
½ papaya and ½ mango	½ papaya and ½ mango

Split the baguette down the middle and spread with Camembert. Add the cranberry sauce and plenty of iceberg lettuce. Peel and seed the papaya, peel and stone the mango, then slice them both and mix together to serve for dessert.

Dinners

Cauliflower Cheese with Green Beans, and Strawberries and Ice Cream

SERVES 4

400 g (14 oz) fresh cauliflower	14 oz fresh cauliflower
480 g (1 lb) new potatoes, scrubbed	1 lb new potatoes, scrubbed
2 tbsp low-fat spread	2 tbsp low-fat spread
25 g (1 oz) flour	¼ cup all-purpose flour
600 ml (1 pint) skimmed milk	2½ cups skim milk
freshly ground black pepper	freshly ground black pepper
pinch of celery salt	pinch of celery salt
100 g (4 oz) reduced-fat Edam cheese, grated	1 cup shredded reduced-fat Edam cheese
360 g (¾ lb) green beans	¾ lb string beans
2 sprigs fresh parsley, chopped	2 sprigs fresh parsley, chopped

440 g (1 lb) strawberries, hulled, washed and halved	1 lb strawberries, hulled, washed and halved
4 x 60 g (2½ oz) scoops ice-cream	4 x 2½ oz scoops ice-cream

Break the cauliflower into florets, cook in a little water, drain and keep warm in a flameproof serving dish.

Put the potatoes on to boil. While they are cooking, make a cheese sauce by melting the low-fat spread in a pan over a medium heat and adding the flour. Stir well for 3 minutes, then remove from the heat and gradually add the milk, stirring all the time. Season to taste with black pepper and celery salt. Stir in the Edam and wait until it has all melted. Pour the cheese sauce over the cauliflower and brown under a hot grill. Also, lightly cook the green beans.

Garnish the cauliflower cheese with the chopped parsley and serve with the potatoes and green beans.

For dessert, serve the strawberries with ice-cream.

Baked Tuna Broccoli

SERVES 4

4 medium baking potatoes	4 medium baking potatoes
180 g (6 oz) tinned tuna in brine, drained and flaked	scant cup drained and flaked canned tuna in brine
180 g (6 oz) tinned sweetcorn, drained	scant cup drained canned sweetcorn
freshly ground black pepper	freshly ground black pepper
pinch of dried mixed herbs	pinch of dried mixed herbs
225 g (½ lb) fresh broccoli florets	½ lb fresh calabrese
150 ml (¼ pint) carrot juice	generous ½ cup carrot juice

340 g (¾ lb) carrots, peeled and sliced	¾ lb carrots, peeled and sliced
200 g (7 oz) mangetout	7 oz snowpeas
25 g (1 oz) wholemeal breadcrumbs	½ cup wholewheat breadcrumbs
20 g (¾ oz) cheese, grated	scant ¼ cup shredded cheese

Pre-heat the oven to 190°C/375°F/gas 5.

Clean the potatoes, prick them with a fork, wrap in foil and bake in the pre-heated oven for 50 minutes, or until cooked through.

Meanwhile, place the flaked tuna in a flameproof and oven-proof dish. Add the sweetcorn and season with pepper and herbs. Cover with the broccoli florets and pour the carrot juice over the top. Cover and bake in the oven for 25 minutes.

Cook the carrots in the meantime and make the topping for the bake. To do this, simply mix the wholemeal breadcrumbs with the cheese. Remove the tuna bake from the oven when it has cooked and sprinkle the breadcrumb mixture over the top. Place under a hot grill for 5 minutes. Meanwhile, cook the mangetout.

Serve the Baked Tuna Broccoli with the potatoes, carrots and mangetout.

Turkey Kebabs

50 g (2 oz) brown rice	¼ cup brown rice
80 g (3 oz) lean turkey, cubed	3 oz lean turkey, cubed
3 cherry tomatoes	3 cherry tomatoes
4 button mushrooms, wiped clean	4 closed mushrooms, wiped clean
¼ yellow pepper, roughly chopped	¼ yellow bell pepper, roughly chopped
1 tbsp lemon juice	1 tbsp lemon juice
freshly ground black pepper	freshly ground black pepper

45 g (1½ oz) Chinese leaves, shredded	¼ cup shredded Napa cabbage
2.5 cm (1 in) chunk cucumber, diced	1 in chunk cucumber, diced
2 tsp fat-free French dressing	2 tsp fat-free French dressing

Put the rice on to cook, following the instructions on the pack.

Meanwhile, thread pieces of turkey, tomatoes, mushrooms and pepper alternately on to skewers. Sprinkle with lemon juice and black pepper and grill for a good 10 minutes, turning every few minutes so that all sides are cooked.

Make a salad from the Chinese leaves, cucumber and dressing and serve with the kebabs and rice.

Skewered Prawns

SERVES 4

2 tbsp olive oil	2 tbsp olive oil
1 tsp chopped fresh thyme	1 tsp chopped fresh thyme
1 tsp chopped fresh dill	1 tsp chopped fresh dill
1 tsp chopped fresh coriander	1 tsp chopped cilantro
salt and freshly ground black pepper	salt and freshly ground black pepper
400 g (14 oz) monkfish, washed and cubed	14 oz monkfish, washed and cubed
24 prawns	24 shrimp
280 g (10 oz) tagliatelle	10 oz tagliatelle
100 g (4 oz) young spinach, washed and shredded	4 oz young spinach, washed and shredded

Mix the olive oil with the chopped fresh herbs and add salt and pepper to taste. Thread cubes of the monkfish and prawns alternately on to skewers. Brush with the oil and herb mix and grill for 5 minutes. Turn, brush again and grill for a further 5 minutes. Use up the oil, basting while cooking if necessary.

Meanwhile, cook the tagliatelle according to the instructions on the pack. Drain, mix it with the spinach and spoon it on to four serving plates. Lay the skewers of fish on the tagliatelle and spinach.

Burger and Salad

55 g (2 oz) very lean minced beef	2 oz very lean ground beef
salt and freshly ground black pepper	salt and freshly ground black pepper
Worcestershire sauce, to taste	Worcestershire sauce, to taste
pinch of dried mixed herbs	pinch of dried mixed herbs
120 g (4½ oz) oven chips	4½ oz oven chips
1 hamburger bun	1 hamburger bun
1 lettuce leaf, washed	1 lettuce leaf, washed
1 tomato, sliced	1 tomato, sliced
4 slices cucumber	4 slices cucumber
ketchup, to serve, if desired	catsup, to serve, if desired

Put the mince in a bowl and season to taste with salt, pepper and a dash of Worcestershire sauce. Add a pinch of mixed herbs and mix well. Form into a burger with your hands and grill both sides until well cooked right through.

Meanwhile, cook the oven chips according to the instructions on the pack. Slice the burger bun and toast the insides until they have just lightly browned.

Place the grilled burger on the bun and add the lettuce, tomato and cucumber. Serve with the oven chips and some ketchup, if you can tolerate it.

Colon-cleansing Recipes

These recipes are designed to bulk up the stools due to their concentration on ingredients containing plenty of insoluble fibre. Remember to drink at least 6 – 8 glasses of water or other fluids every day to keep stools well hydrated. A high-fibre diet minus fluids leads to hard, impacted stools.

Breakfasts

All Bran with Grated Apple

55 g (2 oz) All Bran	scant cup All Bran
1 medium apple, grated	1 medium apple, shredded
150 ml (¼ pint) skimmed milk	½ cup skim milk
1 thick slice granary bread	1 thick slice graham bread
1 tsp low-fat spread	1 tsp low-fat spread
1 tsp marmalade or honey	1 tsp marmalade or honey

Put the All Bran in a bowl and cover with, or mix in, the grated apple. Pour over the skimmed milk and serve.

Toast the bread and serve with the spread and marmalade or honey.

Porridge with Raisins

30 g (1 oz) porridge oats	⅓ cup oatmeal
230 ml (8 fl oz) skimmed milk	1 cup skim milk
2 tsp raisins	2 tsp raisins

2 ready-to-eat apricots	2 ready-to-eat apricots
1 tsp brown sugar	1 tsp brown sugar
1 thick slice wholemeal bread	1 thick slice wholewheat bread
1 tsp low-fat spread	1 tsp low-fat spread
1 tsp marmalade	1 tsp marmalade

Make up the porridge using the skimmed milk according to the instructions on the pack. Once cooked, stir in the raisins and apricots and sprinkle with the brown sugar.

Toast the bread and serve with low-fat spread and marmalade.

Grilled Tomatoes on Toast with Baked Beans

2 slices wholemeal bread	2 slices wholewheat bread
2 tsp low-fat spread	2 tsp low-fat spread
100 g (4 oz) baked beans	1½ cups baked beans
2 tomatoes, halved	2 tomatoes, halved
175 ml (6 fl oz) grapefruit juice, chilled	⅔ cup grapefruit juice, chilled

Toast the bread and spread with the low-fat spread. Heat the beans and spoon on to the toast. Grill the tomato halves and serve with the beans on toast. Have the grapefruit juice with it.

Banana and Date Muffin

1 wholemeal muffin	1 wholewheat muffin
1 medium banana	1 medium banana
1 tbsp chopped dates	1 tbsp chopped dates
2 tsp sesame seeds	2 tsp sesame seeds
grapefruit juice	grapefruit juice

Slice the muffin in half and toast it. Mash the banana with a fork and stir in the chopped dates and the sesame seeds. Spread this mixture over the muffin and serve with a glass of grapefruit juice.

Autumn Cinnamon Compote

SERVES 2

25 g (1 oz) dried apricots	⅛ cup dried apricots
40 g (1½ oz) dried figs	¼ cup dried figs
20 g (¾ oz) dried apples	⅛ cup dried apples
20 g (¾ oz) dried pears	⅛ cup dried pears
20 g (¾ oz) dried peaches	⅛ cup dried peaches
orange juice	orange juice
cinnamon stick	cinnamon stick
2 tbsp low-fat plain yogurt	2 tbsp low-fat plain yogurt
4 tsp toasted sesame seeds	4 tsp toasted sesame seeds

Soak the dried fruit in the orange juice with the cinnamon stick overnight. Place in a saucepan, heat gently and simmer for 15 minutes. Serve hot, topped with the yogurt and sprinkled with the sesame seeds.

Lunches

Lentil Soup with Wholegrain Roll, and Raspberries with Fromage Frais

20 g (8 oz) tinned lentil soup	1 cup canned lentil soup
1 wholegrain roll	1 wholegrain roll
60 g (2½ oz) fresh raspberries or fruit of your choice	½ cup fresh raspberries or fruit of your choice
60 g (2½ oz) plain fromage frais	¼ cup plain fromage blanc

Heat the soup and serve with the roll.

Wash the raspberries and serve in a bowl topped with the fromage frais.

Pizza Muffin

SERVES 2

1 courgette, thinly sliced	1 zucchini, sliced thin
2 plain muffins	2 plain muffins
1 tsp olive oil	1 tsp olive oil
1 garlic clove, crushed	1 garlic clove, crushed
2 tbsp tomato purée	2 tbsp tomato purée
½ red pepper, seeded and cut into strips	½ red pepper, seeded and cut into strips
salt and freshly ground black pepper to taste	salt and freshly ground black pepper to taste
25 g (1 oz) pitted black olives, halved	¼ cup black olives, halved
100 g (3½ oz) reduced-fat cheese, grated	⅔ cup reduced-fat cheese, grated

Cook the sliced courgette in a little boiling water for 1-2 minutes then drain. Split the toast and muffins. Mix the olive oil and garlic together and brush over the toasted muffins. In a bowl, mix together the tomato purée, courgette and red pepper. Season well. Spoon on to the muffins, scatter with the olives and cheese and grill for about 3 minutes, until the cheese is melted and golden.

Hot Salmon Pitta

SERVES 2

200 g (7 oz) tinned salmon drained and flaked	7 oz canned salmon, drained and flaked
2 tbsp mayonnaise	2 tbsp mayonnaise
5 cm piece of cucumber, diced	2 in piece of cucumber, diced
1 spring onion, sliced	1 green onion, sliced
salt and freshly ground black pepper to taste	salt and freshly ground black pepper to taste
2 wholemeal pitta breads	2 wholewheat pitta breads
2 tomatoes, sliced	2 tomatoes, sliced

Mix together the salmon, mayonnaise, cucumber, spring onion and seasoning. Put the pitta breads under a hot grill for a couple of minutes to warm through, then split them and fill with the salmon mixture and sliced tomatoes.

Bean and Pasta Salad

75 g (3 oz) wholemeal macaroni	¾ cup wholewheat macaroni
1 carrot, grated	1 carrot, shredded
1 stick of celery, finely diced	1 stick of celery, finely diced
3 tbsp tinned chickpeas, drained	3 tbsp canned garbanzos, drained
salt and freshly ground black pepper	salt and freshly ground black pepper
½ small pot of plain yogurt	½ small pot of plain yogurt
2 sprigs fresh parsley, chopped, to garnish	2 sprigs fresh parsley, chopped, to garnish
1 orange	1 orange

Cook the macaroni according to the instructions on the pack. Drain and leave to cool.

Stir the carrot, celery and chickpeas into the cooled macaroni. Season to taste, then mix in the yogurt. Sprinkle the parsley over and serve.

Have the orange for dessert.

Cottage Coleslaw

100 g (4 oz) white cabbage, shredded	1 cup shredded white cabbage
1 medium courgette, grated	1 medium zucchini, shredded
1 orange, peeled and chopped	1 orange, peeled and chopped
100 g (4 oz) cottage cheese	½ cup cottage cheese
2 tbsp low-fat plain yogurt	2 tbsp low-fat plain yogurt
freshly ground black pepper	freshly ground black pepper
1 pitta bread	1 pitta bread

Mix together the cabbage and courgette. Add the orange and cottage cheese and stir in the yogurt. Season with the black pepper to taste. Cut the pitta bread in half crossways to make two individual pockets. Use the Cottage Coleslaw mixture to fill the pitta pockets.

Dinners

Poussin/Cornish Game Hen Grilled with Lime and Coriander

A simple marinade flavours and protects the poussin from the heat of the grill. Lemon or orange can be substituted for the lime, or you can use dry white wine. This dish is perfect for summer barbecues.

SERVES 2

grated rind and juice of 2 limes	grated rind and juice of 2 limes
grated rind of 1 lemon	grated rind of 1 lemon
2 tbsp olive oil	2 tbsp olive oil
4 shallots or 1 small onion, very finely chopped	4 scallions or 1 small onion, very finely chopped
1 tbsp chopped fresh coriander	1 tbsp chopped fresh cilantro
salt and freshly ground black pepper to taste	salt and freshly ground black pepper to taste
2 spatchcocked poussins	2 Cornish game hens
300 g (10 oz) carrots, sliced	2 cups carrots, sliced
120 g (3 oz) brown rice	⅔ cup brown rice
fresh coriander leaves, to garnish	fresh cilantro leaves, to garnish

Preheat the grill to medium. Mix the grated lime and lemon rind with the lime juice and olive oil, then stir in the shallots or onion, chopped coriander and black pepper. Slash the poussins' breasts and legs at 2.5cm intervals and rub the marinade all over the birds. Cover and leave to marinate, turning occasionally, for 3-4 hours.

Place the birds, skin-side uppermost, 10cm from the grill and cook for 20-30 minutes, turning twice, until the skin is crisp and golden and the juices run clear when the meat is pierced at the thickest part. Meanwhile, cook the carrots in a little water until tender, then drain, purée and season to taste. Cook the rice and serve with the poussins and the carrot purée. Garnish with coriander leaves.

Stir-fried Duck with Noodles

Duck can be fatty, but if you remove the skin and visible fat this is greatly reduced. A lot of the fat is the monounsaturated type, which is an important part of any healthy diet.

SERVES 4

4 duck breasts (150 g (6 oz) each), skin and fat removed	4 duck breasts (6 oz) each, skin and fat removed
¼ tsp ground ginger	¼ tsp ground ginger
2 shallots, finely chopped	2 scallions, finely chopped
2 cloves garlic, crushed	2 cloves garlic, crushed
2 tsp coriander seeds, finely crushed	2 tsp coriander seeds, finely crushed
juice of ½ lemon	juice of ½ lemon
240 g (8 oz) rice	1⅛ cups rice
2 tbsp oil	2 tbsp oil
250 g (8 oz) mangetout topped, tailed and cut into strips	2 cups snow peas, topped, tailed and cut into strips
200 g (7 oz) carrots, cut into thin strips	1½ cups carrots, cut into thin strips
90 ml (3 fl oz) dry red wine	⅓ cup dry red wine
180 ml (6 fl oz) chicken stock	¾ cup chicken stock
salt and freshly ground black pepper to taste	salt and freshly ground black pepper to taste
1 tsp cornflour	1 tsp cornflour
½ pomegranate	½ pomegranate
140g (5½ oz) cooked wholegrain noodles	1 cup cooked wholegrain noodles

Cut the duck breasts into thin strips and put them into a bowl with the ginger, shallots, garlic, coriander seeds and lemon juice. Cover and leave to marinate for 1 hour.

Cook the rice in plenty of boiling salted water until just tender then drain thoroughly. Meanwhile, heat the oil in a large frying pan or wok, add the duck and its marinade and stir-fry for 5 minutes. Add the mangetout and carrot strips and continue to cook for 2 minutes then pour in the wine and stock and simmer for 2 minutes. Season to taste.

Blend the cornflour with a little water, stir into the pan with the pomegranate kernels and heat until the sauce thickens. Serve with the rice.

Serve with the noodles, cooked according to the directions on the pack and drained.

Vegetable Couscous

SERVES 2

2 tbsp olive oil	2 tbsp olive oil
1 onion, chopped	1 onion, chopped
1 clove garlic, crushed	1 clove garlic, minced
1 tsp tomato purée	1 tsp tomato paste
salt and freshly ground black pepper	salt and freshly ground black pepper
pinch of cumin	pinch of cumin
pinch of turmeric	pinch of turmeric
pinch of paprika	pinch of paprika
pinch of ground coriander	pinch of ground coriander
pinch of ground ginger	pinch of ground ginger
1 tsp chilli sauce	1 tsp chili sauce
300 ml (½ pint) water	1¼ cups water
1 carrot, sliced	1 carrot, sliced
1 potato, diced	1 potato, diced
55 g (2 oz) turnip, diced	⅓ cup diced turnip
1 tomato, chopped	1 tomato, chopped
1 courgette, sliced	1 zucchini, sliced
200 g (7 oz) tinned chickpeas, drained	1½ cups drained canned garbanzos
100 g (4 oz) instant couscous	⅔ cup instant couscous
60 g (2½ oz) raspberries	½ cup raspberries
100 g (4 oz) strawberries, hulled, washed and halved	scant cup strawberries, hulled, washed and halved
4 tbsp Greek yogurt	4 tbsp Greek yogurt

Heat the oil in a large pan and add the onion and garlic. Cook for a few minutes, stirring well until softened. Add the tomato purée, a pinch each of salt and pepper, the cumin, turmeric, paprika, coriander, ginger and chilli sauce. Pour in half the water, cover, bring to the boil and simmer for 15 minutes.

Add the carrot, potato and turnip. Cover and cook for a further 30 minutes.

Add the tomato, courgette and chickpeas. Adjust the seasoning to taste if necessary and cook for 15 minutes more.

Meanwhile, make up the couscous according to the instructions on the pack. Serve with the vegetables.

For dessert, serve the raspberries and strawberries mixed together, each portion topped with a spoonful of Greek yogurt.

Grilled Cod with Baked Pumpkin and Ginger

SERVES 2

450 g (16 oz) pumpkin, peeled, seeds removed, and cut into chunks	3¼ cups pumpkin, peeled, seeds removed, and cut into chunks
25 g (1 oz) stem ginger and 150 ml (5 fl oz) ginger syrup from the jar	¼ cup ginger and ⅔ cup ginger syrup from the jar
2 oranges	2 oranges
salt and freshly ground black pepper to taste	salt and freshly ground black pepper to taste
1 tbsp sunflower oil	1 tbsp sunflower oil
2 cod fillets, about 175 g each	2 cod fillets, about 175 g each
grated rind of ½ lemon	grated rind of ½ lemon
150 ml (5 fl oz) white wine	⅔ cup white wine
pinch of paprika	pinch of paprika
200 g wholemeal pasta, to serve	2 cups wholewheat pasta, to serve

Boil the pumpkin for 7 minutes, drain and place in an ovenproof dish. Finely chop the ginger and sprinkle over the pumpkin. Grate the rind from the oranges, then remove all the peel and divide the oranges into segments. Sprinkle the rind over the pumpkin, together with the seasoning, oil and ginger syrup. Bake at 200°C/ 400°F/Gas Mark 6 for 35-40 minutes.

Meanwhile place the fish in a bowl with the lemon rind, wine, paprika and seasoning and leave to marinate while the pumpkin is baking, then grill for about 8 minutes either side. Cook the pasta until *al dente* then drain. Serve the fish with the pumpkin, garnished with the orange segments, and accompanied by the pasta.

Bean Casserole

SERVES 4

50 g (2 oz) dried black-eyed beans	¼ cup dried black-eyed beans
50 g (2 oz) dried butter beans	¼ cup dried lima beans
50 g (2 oz) dried haricot beans	¼ cup dried navy beans
50 g (2 oz) dried red kidney beans	heaped ¼ cup dried red kidney beans
4 tomatoes, chopped	4 tomatoes, chopped
1 green pepper, seeded and chopped	1 green bell pepper, seeded and chopped
50 g (2 oz) mushrooms, wiped and sliced	1 cup wiped, sliced mushrooms
2 tbsp chopped fresh coriander	2 tbsp chopped cilantro
2 cloves	2 cloves
2 tbsp clear honey	2 tbsp clear honey
1 tbsp wine vinegar	1 tbsp wine vinegar

| salt and freshly ground black pepper | salt and freshly ground black pepper |
| 240 g (9 oz) brown rice | 1¼ cups brown rice |

Soak all the beans, except the red kidney beans, in plenty of water overnight. Soak the red kidney beans in a separate bowl, also overnight.

Next day, drain the red kidney beans, change the water and boil rapidly for a full 10 minutes. Drain and rinse all the beans, then cook all of them together for 1 hour in fresh water until tender.

Then stir in the tomatoes, green pepper, mushrooms, coriander and cloves. Add the honey and wine vinegar and season to taste with salt and pepper. Simmer for a further 30 minutes. Meanwhile, cook the rice, then serve with the casserole.

Lactose-free Recipes

These recipes are for people who cannot tolerate the milk sugar known as lactose. Soy milk has been substituted for cow's milk in some recipes.

Breakfasts

Porridge with Sunflower Seeds

200 ml (7 fl oz) water or soya milk	¾ cup water or soya milk
75 g (3 oz) porridge oats	1 cup porridge oats
1 tbsp honey-roasted sunflower seeds	1 tbsp honey-roasted sunflower seeds
glass of orange juice to serve	glass of orange juice to serve

Pour the milk into a small saucepan, add the porridge oats and bring slowly to a boil. Simmer for a few minutes to thicken, stirring constantly, then pour into a bowl. Sprinkle with the sunflower seeds and serve with the orange juice.

Citrus Fruit Cup with Peanut Butter Crumpets

Peanut butter is a useful source of vitamin E and protein. Since it is also high in fat it is a good idea to have it instead of, rather than as well as, butter or margarine.

1 small grapefruit	1 small grapefruit
1 small orange	1 small orange
2 crumpets	2 crumpets or 1 English muffin, halved
tbsp peanut butter	tbsp peanut butter

Peel and slice the grapefruit and orange then mix them together in a bowl. Chill before serving. Follow the fruit cup with the crumpets, toasted and spread with crunchy peanut butter.

Apple and Almond Muesli/Granola with Soya Milk

50 g (2 oz) muesli (check label)	½ cup granola
2 tsp toasted flaked almonds	2 tsp toasted flaked almonds
1 apple, grated	1 apple, grated
1 kiwi fruit, peeled and chopped	1 kiwi fruit, peeled and chopped
150 ml (5 fl oz) soya milk	⅔ cup soya milk

Mix the muesli with the toasted almonds. Top with the grated apple and the kiwi fruit then pour over the milk to serve.

Poached Eggs on Toast

2 slices of granary bread	2 slices of graham bread
1 egg	1 egg
2 tomatoes	2 tomatoes
milk-free margarine	milk-free margarine
200 ml (7 fl oz) glass of pink grapefruit juice	¾ cup glass of pink grapefruit juice

Toast the bread and cut it into triangles. Poach the egg and grill the tomatoes. Spread the toast lightly with sunflower margarine and top with the egg and tomatoes. Serve with the grapefruit juice.

Crispy Bacon and Tomato Baguette

2 rashers lean back bacon	2 slices lean bacon strips
large chunk of granary stick	large chunk of French or Italian bread
2 tsp milk-free margarine	2 tsp milk-free margarine
1 large tomato, sliced	1 large tomato, sliced

Grill the bacon until crisp then dice it. Heat the bread in the oven and split it open lengthways. Spread one side with the butter, then make a sandwich with the grilled bacon and sliced tomato.

Lunches

Carrot Soup

1 tsp oil	1tsp oil
2 carrots, chopped	2 carrots, chopped
1 small leek, trimmed and finely chopped	1 small leek, trimmed and finely chopped

250–300 ml (8–10 fl oz) vegetable stock	¾–1⅓ cup vegetable stock

salt and freshly ground
  black pepper to taste
	salt and freshly ground
	  black pepper to taste

handful of chopped fresh
  coriander or parsley
	handful of chopped fresh
	  cilantro or parsley

homemade wholemeal scone, to serve	wholewheat roll, to serve

Heat the oil in a small pan, add the carrots and leek and cook gently for a few minutes. Pour in the stock, season and bring to the boil, then reduce the heat, cover and simmer for 15–20 minutes. Add the coriander or parsley, transfer the mixture to a blender or food processor and purée. Return the soup to the pan to heat through and serve with the wholemeal scone.

Avocado Dip with Rice Cakes

1 small avocado	1 small avocado
1 tbsp lemon juice	1 tbsp lemon juice

hot pepper sauce, such
  as Tabasco
	hot pepper sauce, such
	  as Tabasco

salt and freshly ground
  black pepper to taste
	salt and freshly ground
	  black pepper to taste

2 carrots	2 carrots
3 rice cakes	3 rice cakes

5 no-need-to-soak dried
  apricots, or fresh apricots,
  for dessert
	5 no-need-to-soak dried
	  apricots, or fresh apricots,
	  for dessert

Peel and stone the avocado then mash the flesh with the lemon juice, hot pepper sauce and seasoning. Peel the carrots and cut them into batons. Serve the avocado dip with the carrots and rice cakes, and have the apricots for dessert.

Mackerel Rice Pot

50 g (2 oz) cooked brown rice (un-cooked weight)	¼ cup cooked brown rice (uncooked weight)
2 spring onions, chopped	2 green onions, chopped
1 tbsp chopped fresh basil	1 tbsp chopped fresh basil
¼ green pepper, chopped	¼ green pepper, chopped
75 g (3 oz) mackerel, canned in tomato sauce	3oz mackerel, canned in tomato sauce
2 tbsp reduced-fat mayonnaise (check label)	2 tbsp reduced-fat mayonnaise (check label)
dash of Worcestershire sauce	dash of Worcestershire sauce
1 large apple, for dessert	1 large apple, for dessert

Mix together the rice, spring onions, basil, green pepper, mackerel, mayonnaise and Worcestershire sauce. Serve followed by a large apple for dessert.

Mini Niçoise

SERVES 2

lettuce leaves	lettuce leaves
1 potato, cooked and diced	1 potato, cooked and diced
1 small tin tuna, drained and flaked	1 small can tuna, drained and flaked
2 small eggs, hard boiled, shelled and sliced	2 size-3 eggs, hard boiled, shelled and sliced
½ green pepper, seeded and cut into strips	½ green pepper, seeded and cut into strips
2 tbsp green beans, lightly cooked	2 tbsp string beans, lightly cooked
2 tomatoes, chopped	2 tomatoes, chopped

25 g (1 oz) black olives	¼ cup black olives
4 anchovy fillets (optional)	2 anchovies, chopped (optional)
1 tbsp vinaigrette dressing	1 tbsp vinaigrette dressing
2 wholemeal rolls	2 wholewheat rolls

Make a bed of lettuce on 2 plates then arrange the potato, tuna, egg, green pepper, beans and tomatoes over it. Top with the olives and anchovy, if using, and drizzle with a little vinaigrette.

BLT Open Sandwich

Here is a way of transforming a normally 'unhealthy' sandwich into one that conforms to healthy eating guidelines. Make sure you use lean bacon and reduced-calorie mayonnaise.

SERVES 2

4 rashers lean smoked back bacon, fat removed	4 slices lean smoked bacon, strips, fat removed
4 slices of French bread	4 slices of French bread
2 tsp reduced-calorie mayonnaise (check label)	2 tsp reduced-calorie mayonnaise (check label)
2 large tomatoes, sliced	2 large tomatoes, sliced
1 little Gem lettuce, shredded	4 lettuce leaves, shredded
salt and freshly ground black pepper to taste	salt and freshly ground black pepper to taste

Grill the bacon and lightly toast the bread. Spread the mayonnaise on the toast, place the bacon on top then arrange the tomatoes and lettuce on top of that. Season well and serve.

Dinners

Mixed Herb Omelette

1–2 tbsp chopped fresh
   mixed herbs, such as
   parsley, chives and tarragon
2 eggs
salt and freshly ground
   black pepper to taste
2 tsp sunflower oil
2 cherry tomatoes, halved
1 large tomato, quartered
crusty caraway seed bread,
   to serve

1–2 tbsp chopped fresh
   mixed herbs, such as
   parsley, chives and tarragon
2 eggs
salt and freshly ground
   black pepper to taste
2 tsp sunflower oil
2 cherry tomatoes, halved
1 large tomato, quartered
crusty caraway seed bread,
   to serve

Put the herbs, eggs and seasoning together into a bowl and beat lightly until combined. Heat the oil in a small frying pan and pour in the egg mixture. Keep lifting the edges with a fork so the uncooked egg on top runs underneath, then when the centre is just set, turn the omelette out on to a plate. Mix the tomatoes together, season and serve with the omelette, along with a chunk of crusty caraway seed bread.

Chinese Spinach and Pine Nuts with Noodles

SERVES 4

900 g (32 oz) fresh young
   spinach
600 g (21 oz) plain noodles
100 g (4 oz) mushrooms,
   finely sliced
1 tbsp sesame oil

16 cups fresh young spinach

7 cups plain noodles
1¼ cups mushrooms,
   finely sliced
1 tbsp sesame oil

¼ tsp Chinese five-spice powder	¼ tsp Chinese five-spice powder
1 tbsp light soy sauce	1 tbsp light soy sauce
1 large tbsp pine nuts	1 large tbsp pine nuts

Remove any tough stalks from the spinach and wash the leaves very thoroughly. Place in a large pan with just the water that clings to the leaves, then cover and cool gently until the leaves have wilted. Drain well, then arrange in a serving dish and keep hot.

Cook the noodles, according to the directions on the packet. Quickly saute the mushrooms in the oil until softened. Stir in the five-spice powder, soy sauce and pine nuts and stir-fry for 1 minute. Spoon over the spinach and serve immediately with the noodles.

Barbecued Seafood Kebabs

SERVES 4

5 limes	5 limes
1 red chilli, chopped	1 red chilli, chopped
1 tbsp oil, plus extra for brushing	1 tbsp oil, plus extra for brushing
salt and freshly ground black pepper to taste	salt and freshly ground black pepper to taste
8 large peeled prawns	8 peeled jumbo shrimp
700 g (24 oz) firm white fish fillets such as monkfish or cod, skinned and cut into 2.5 cm cubes	4 cups firm white fish such as cod, skinned and cut into 1 in cubes.
1 yellow pepper, seeded and chopped	1 yellow pepper, seeded and chopped
240 g (9 oz) brown rice	1¼ cups brown rice

Grate the rind and squeeze the juice from 2 of the limes, and put into a dish with the chopped chilli, oil and salt and pepper. Add the prawns and white fish, toss to coat with the marinade, then cover and refrigerate for 1 hour.

Cut each remaining lime into 8 wedges and arrange on 8 skewers with the fish cubes, prawns and the yellow pepper. Cook the rice in plenty of boiling salted water until just tender then drain. Meanwhile, brush the kebabs with oil and cook on a prepared barbecue or under a medium-hot grill for 6–10 minutes, turning once and brushing with the marinade. Serve with the rice.

Moroccan Spring Lamb

Lamb can be fatty, so it's best to trim off the visible fat. There'll still be some in the flesh to add flavour.

SERVES 2

250 g (9 oz) lamb fillet, all visible fat removed, cut into large cubes	1⅛ cups lamb fillet, all visible fat removed, cut into large cubes
1 tsp ground cinnamon	1 tsp ground cinnamon
2 onions, sliced	2 onions, sliced
100 g (3½ oz) no-need-to-soak dried prunes, halved	½ cup dried prunes, halved
300 ml (10 fl oz) lamb or vegetable stock	1⅓ cups lamb or vegetable stock
200 g (6½ oz) boiled potatoes	1⅓ cups boiled potatoes
spring greens	collard greens

Heat a heavy-based pan, add the lamb and the cinnamon and fry for 1 minute. Stir in the onions, prunes and stock. Bring to the boil then cover, reduce the heat and simmer for about 30 minutes until the meat is tender. Serve with steamed spring greens and boiled potatoes.

Chicken Breasts with Raspberries

SERVES 4

600 g (20 oz) potatoes, to serve	4 cups potatoes, to serve
4 skinned, boned chicken breasts (120 g (4 oz) each)	4 skinned, boned chicken breasts (4 oz each)
2 tbsp plain flour	2 tbsp plain flour
1 tbsp olive oil	1 tbsp olive oil
4 tbsp raspberry vinegar	4 tbsp raspberry vinegar
2 tbsp redcurrant jelly	2 tbsp red currant or cranberry sauce
4 tbsp port	4 tbsp port
salt and white pepper	salt and white pepper
100 g (4 oz) fresh raspberries	1 cup fresh raspberries

Peel the potatoes and cook them in boiling salted water until tender, then drain and mash. Meanwhile, toss the chicken breasts in the flour then heat the oil in a pan and fry the chicken for about 4 minutes per side, until golden brown. Remove the chicken from the pan and keep warm. Deglaze the pan juices with the raspberry vinegar then add the redcurrant jelly and the port. Stir together and boil rapidly until the sauce thickens. Season to taste. Just before serving, add the fresh raspberries to the sauce. Pour the sauce over the chicken and serve with the mashed potatoes.

Wheat-free Recipes

Some people cannot tolerate wheat in their diets because it causes, among other things, bloating and abdominal discomfort. These recipes are wheat-free but not gluten-free (gluten is present in wheat, barley, oats and rye), and should not be used by people with coeliac disease.

Breakfasts

Strawberry Special K and Rye Bread Toast

150 ml (¼ pint) semi-skimmed milk	⅔ cup semi-skim milk
40 g (1⅛ oz) Special K	1 cup Special K
5–6 strawberries sliced, or fruit of your choice	5–6 strawberries sliced, or fruit of your choice
1 slice fresh rye bread	1 slice fresh rye bread
butter	butter
Marmite	yeast extract

Mix the fruit in a bowl with the Special K and serve with the milk. Toast the rye bread and serve with butter and Marmite.

Fruit Kebabs

SERVES 2

1 small banana	1 small banana
1 apple	1 apple
1 orange	1 orange
1 kiwi fruit	1 kiwi fruit
2 poppyseed rye crispbreads	2 poppyseed rye crispbreads or crackers
1 tbsp low-fat cream cheese	1 tbsp low-fat cream cheese

Peel the fruit where necessary then chop it into neat cubes and thread it on to skewers. Serve accompanied by the crispbreads, spread with cream cheese.

Mango Shake

Mangoes are rich in beta-carotene, so are a particularly good fruit to use in this shake, but you can substitute nectarines or peaches if you prefer.

1 medium-sized ripe mango, peeled, stoned and cubed	1 medium-sized ripe mango, peeled, stoned and cubed
250 ml (8 fl oz) semi-skimmed milk	1 cup semi-skim milk
150 g (5 oz) low-fat plain yogurt	⅔ cup low-fat plain yogurt
mint sprigs to garnish	mint sprigs to garnish

Purée the mango in a blender with the milk and yogurt. Chill if time allows, then serve garnished with mint sprigs.

Quick Kedgeree

Having a fish dish such as this for breakfast is a filling way to start the day.

50 g (2 oz) easy-cook rice	¼ cup easy-cook rice
1 tbsp peas	1 tbsp peas
75 g (3 oz) smoked haddock	3 oz smoked haddock
25 g (1 oz) mushrooms	⅓ cup mushrooms
2 tbsp low-fat plain yogurt	2 tbsp low-fat plain yogurt
1 tsp curry paste	1 tsp curry paste
salt and freshly ground black pepper to taste	salt and freshly ground black pepper to taste
large chunk of 100% rye bread	large chunk of 100% rye bread
glass of ruby-red orange juice, to serve	glass of ruby-red orange juice, to serve

Cook the rice in boiling salted water until just tender, adding the peas for the last few minutes. Drain and set aside. Lightly poach the smoked haddock, then drain and flake it. Grill the mushrooms and chop them. Blend the yogurt with the curry paste.

Mix together the rice and peas, haddock, mushrooms and seasoning to taste then stir in the yogurt. Warm through in a low oven, then serve with the bread and the orange juice.

Instant Oat Cereal with Apple and Toast

40 g (1½ oz) instant porridge	½ cup instant oatmeal
175 ml (6 fl oz) skimmed milk	⅔ cup skim milk
2 tbsp sweetened stewed apple	2 tbsp applesauce
1 tsp raisins	1 tsp raisins
1 slice 100% rye bread	1 slice 100% rye bread
1 tsp low-fat spread	1 tsp low-fat spread
1 tsp honey	1 tsp honey

Make up the cereal, warming the milk, as directed on the pack. Serve with the apple and raisins. Toast the bread and serve with the low-fat spread and honey.

Lunches

Yellow Pepper Soup with Rye Bread

Peppers are one of the richest vegetable sources of vitamin C, and carrots are among the richest sources of beta-carotene, so this soup is bursting with goodness.

SERVES 2

2 yellow peppers, seeded
  and chopped
2 potatoes, chopped
4 carrots, chopped
salt and freshly ground
  black pepper to taste
2 100% rye bread rolls, to serve

2 yellow peppers, seeded
  and chopped
2 potatoes, chopped
4 carrots, chopped
salt and freshly ground
  black pepper to taste
2 100% rye bread rolls, to serve

Put 450ml water in a large pan, add the peppers, potatoes, carrots and seasoning and simmer for 20 minutes or until the vegetables are tender. Cool the soup slightly, then purée in a blender or food processor. Return to the pan and heat through. Taste and adjust the seasoning, then serve with the hot rolls.

Apricot, Almond and Orange Rice Pot

SERVES 2

6 dried apricots, chopped
1 large orange, peeled and
  cut into segments
200 g (7 oz) cooked brown
  rice (cooked weight)
50 g (2 oz) almonds,
  roughly chopped
salt and freshly ground
  black pepper to taste
1 tbsp lemon juice
2 tsp chopped fresh parsley

6 dried apricots, chopped
1 large orange, peeled and
  cut into segments
1¼ cups cooked brown
  rice (cooked weight)
½ cup almonds,
  roughly chopped
salt and freshly ground
  black pepper to taste
1 tbsp lemon juice
2 tsp chopped fresh parsley

Toss the apricots and orange segments together with the rice and almonds. Season to taste, then sprinkle with the lemon juice and parsley.

Baked Sweet Potatoes with Stilton

Sweet potatoes are the best single source of all three antioxidant vitamins. The ones with orange-coloured flesh contain more beta-carotene than their paler counterparts. This recipe makes a change from ordinary baked potatoes.

SERVES 4

4 large sweet potatoes	4 large sweet potatoes
a little oil	a little oil
salt and freshly ground black pepper to taste	salt and freshly ground black pepper to taste
115 g (4½ oz) Stilton cheese, grated or crumbled	1 cup Stilton cheese, grated or crumbled
150 g (6 oz) low-fat fromage frais	⅔ cup low-fat fromage frais
50 g (1 oz) iceberg lettuce, finely shredded	½ cup iceberg lettuce, finely shredded
finely chopped fresh parsley, to garnish	finely chopped fresh parsley, to garnish

Wipe the potatoes with a damp cloth, rub the skins with a little oil and then with a little salt. Prick each potato three or four times and bake in the oven at 200°C/400°F/Gas Mark 6 for 1 hour or until tender. Split each potato in half lengthways, and scoop most of the flesh into a bowl; mash, and then mix in just over half the Stilton, all the fromage frais, lettuce, and salt and pepper to taste. Spoon the mixture back into each potato skin and sprinkle with the remaining Stilton. Return to the oven for a further 5–10 minutes until the cheese has melted and the filling is hot. Serve sprinkled with chopped parsley.

Spinach and Red Pepper Omelette

½ red pepper	½ red pepper
90 g (3½ oz) fresh spinach	2 cups fresh spinach
1 clove garlic, crushed (optional)	1 clove garlic, crushed (optional)
1 tsp olive oil	1 tsp olive oil
chopped fresh parsley	chopped fresh parsley
salt and freshly ground black pepper to taste	salt and freshly ground black pepper to taste
2 eggs	2 eggs
2 tbsp milk	2 tbsp milk
2 rye crispbreads	2 rye crispbreads

For dessert

1 kiwi fruit, peeled and sliced	1 kiwi fruit, peeled and sliced
small bunch of green grapes	small bunch of green grapes
1 Granny Smith apple, cored and chopped	1 Granny Smith apple, cored and chopped
squeeze of lemon juice	squeeze of lemon juice

Cut the red pepper half into 2 and place the pieces under a pre-heated grill. Cook until the skin is charred and blistered in places, then leave to cool slightly. Peel off the skin and cut the red pepper into strips.

Heat the olive oil in a small frying pan then saute the spinach, and the garlic if using, for a few minutes until wilted. Mix in the red pepper strips, parsley and seasoning. Lightly beat together the eggs and milk then pour this mixture over the vegetables and cook over a gentle heat until the omelette is set and lightly browned underneath. Place the omelette under a hot grill for a few minutes to finish cooking the top then turn out on to a plate. Serve cold, cut into wedges, and accompanied by the crispbread.

Finish lunch with a green fruit salad made by mixing together the kiwi fruit, grapes, apple and a squeeze of lemon juice.

Sweet Potato Salad

1 large sweet potato	1 large sweet potato
1 egg, hard-boiled, shelled and chopped	1 egg, hard-boiled, shelled and chopped
1 tomato, chopped	1 tomato, chopped
2 tbsp mayonnaise	2 tbsp mayonnaise
salt and freshly ground black pepper to taste	salt and freshly ground black pepper to taste
Chinese leaves	bok choy leaves
1 orange or other citrus fruit, for dessert	1 orange or other citrus fruit, for dessert

Cook the sweet potato in boiling salted water until tender then drain. When cool enough to handle, peel and cut into chunks. Mix the hard-boiled egg and the tomato with the mayonnaise, season well, then stir in the potato chunks. Serve on a bed of Chinese leaves and follow with an orange or other citrus fruit for dessert.

Dinners

Stuffed Aubergines/Eggplant

SERVES 2

2 medium aubergines	2 medium eggplant
2 tbsp sunflower oil	2 tbsp sunflower oil
1 onion, chopped	1 onion, chopped
225 g (8 oz) cooked lentils (cooked weight)	1¼ cups cooked lentils (cooked weight)
3–4 tbsp chopped fresh parsley	3–4 tbsp chopped fresh parsley
½ tsp finely grated lemon rind	½ tsp finely grated lemon rind
1 clove garlic, crushed	1 clove garlic, crushed
1 large tomato, chopped	1 large tomato, chopped
175 g (6 oz) cooked brown rice (cooked weight)	1 cup cooked brown rice (cooked weight)
salt and freshly ground black pepper to taste	salt and freshly ground black pepper to taste
2 tbsp grated cheese	2 tbsp grated cheese
twists of lemon, to garnish	twists of lemon, to garnish

Cut the aubergines in half lengthways and scoop out the flesh to within 1 cm of the skins. Chop the flesh. Blanch the aubergine shells in boiling water for 2 minutes then drain well.

Heat the oil and fry the aubergine flesh and the onion until soft. Add the lentils and cook for 3–4 minutes, then stir in all the remaining ingredients except the cheese and lemon twists. Stuff the aubergine shells with this mixture, cover and bake in the oven at 200°C/400°F/Gas Mark 6 for 15–20 minutes. Serve hot, garnished with a sprinkling of cheese and the lemon twists.

Celery and Tomato Gratin

SERVES 4

1 medium head of celery, cut into 5 cm lengths	1 medium head of celery, cut into 2 in lengths
1 large onion, finely chopped	1 large onion, finely chopped
1 clove garlic, crushed	1 clove garlic, crushed
3 tbsp olive oil	3 tbsp olive oil
450 g (16 oz) tomatoes, skinned, seeded and chopped	2 cups tomatoes, skinned, seeded and chopped
½ tsp caster sugar	½ tsp finely granulated sugar
6 tbsp dry white wine or cider	6 tbsp dry white wine or cider
salt and freshly ground black pepper to taste	salt and freshly ground black pepper to taste
16 pitted black olives	16 pitted black olives
50 g (1½ oz) Gruyère cheese, grated	¾ cup Gruyère cheese, grated
280 g (10 oz) rice	1½ cups rice

Put the celery into a saucepan with enough water just to cover, and bring to the boil. Simmer gently until just tender, then drain. Meanwhile, gently fry the onion and garlic in the oil for 3–4 minutes. Add the tomatoes, sugar, wine or cider, and salt and pepper to taste. Simmer gently for 15 minutes.

Put the cooked celery into a greased ovenproof dish. Scatter the olives over the top then pour over the tomato sauce and sprinkle with the grated cheese. Bake in the oven at 200°C/400°F/Gas Mark 6 for 15 minutes. Cook the rice in plenty of boiling salted water until tender then drain and serve with the gratin.

Egg Tatties

SERVES 2

2 large baking potatoes
3 eggs
1 tbsp semi-skimmed milk
salt and freshly ground
    black pepper to taste
1 tsp butter
1 tbsp chopped fresh chives
2 tbsp low-fat plain yogurt
crisp lettuce leaves and
    ½ green pepper, chopped,
    to serve

Wash the potatoes and prick the skins at regular intervals, then wrap them in foil and bake in the oven at 200°C/400°F/Gas Mark 6 for 1¼ hours, until tender.

Just before the potatoes are ready, beat the eggs with the milk and salt and pepper. Melt the butter in a small pan and stir in the eggs. Scramble lightly over a gentle heat until the eggs form soft creamy curds. Halve each potato lengthways and scoop out the flesh. Mash the potato flesh and mix lightly with the scrambled egg, chives and yogurt. Spoon back into the potato shells, cover loosely with foil and return to the oven for another 4–5 minutes. Serve with the lettuce and green pepper.

Caribbean Fish Stew

Packed with peppers, this dish is just bursting with vitamin C.

SERVES 4

250 g (8 oz) unpeeled prawns	2 cups unpeeled jumbo shrimp
1 bay leaf	1 bay leaf
1 slice of lemon	1 slice of lemon
2 cloves garlic, crushed	2 cloves garlic, crushed
grated rind and juice of 1 lime	grated rind and juice of 1 lime
1 tsp chopped fresh ginger root	1 tsp chopped fresh ginger root
350 g (12 oz) fresh tuna or swordfish, skinned and cubed	12 oz fresh tuna or swordfish, skinned and cubed
250 g (12 oz) thick cod steak, skinned and cubed	12 oz thick cod steak, skinned and cubed
320 g (10 oz) brown rice	1½ cups brown rice
2 tbsp oil	2 tbsp oil
1 small onion, finely chopped	1 small onion, finely chopped
1 red and 1 green pepper, seeded and diced	1 red and 1 green pepper, seeded and diced
120 ml (4 fl oz) dry white wine	½ cup dry white wine
1 tsp demerara sugar	1 tsp brown sugar
1 small mango, peeled, stoned and diced	1 small mango, peeled, stoned and diced
½ small pineapple, peeled, cored and chopped	½ small pineapple, peeled, cored and chopped
salt and freshly ground black pepper to taste	salt and freshly ground black pepper to taste
2 tsp cornflour	2 tsp cornflour

Peel the prawns, put the shells into a saucepan, and refrigerate the prawns until needed. Add the bay leaf and lemon to the pan, cover the shells with water and bring to the boil. Simmer for 30 minutes. Meanwhile, put the garlic, lime rind and juice, and ginger into a dish, add the fish, toss together and marinate for 30 minutes. Cook the brown rice in plenty of boiling salted water until tender, then drain. Strain the prawn stock into a jug, return to a clean pan and boil until reduced to 150ml. Heat the oil in a large saucepan, add the onion and peppers and cook for 5 minutes over a medium heat. Add the reduced stock, the marinade (but not the fish) and the wine and sugar, and simmer for 15 minutes.

Stir in the cubes of fish and cook for 5 minutes then blend the cornflour with 1 tablespoon of water and stir it into the stew. Add the mango, pineapple and peeled prawns and cook for 3–4 minutes, until thickened. Taste, and season if necessary. Serve with the brown rice.

Pork and Lentil Casserole

Pork can be almost as lean as chicken, and is just as versatile. In this simple casserole it is combined with carrots, one of the best sources of beta-carotene.

SERVES 4

4 large baking potatoes, to serve	4 large baking potatoes, to serve
250 g (8 oz) carrots, cut into chunks	1½ cups carrots, cut into chunks
1 large courgette, cut into chunks	1 large zucchini, cut into chunks
100 g (4 oz) mushrooms, quartered	1¼ cups mushrooms, quartered
1 tbsp olive oil	1 tbsp olive oil

500 g (18 oz) lean boneless pork, cut into cubes	2¼ cups lean boneless pork, cut into cubes
1 medium onion, sliced	1 medium onion, sliced
salt and freshly ground black pepper to taste	salt and freshly ground black pepper to taste
50 g (1¾ oz) brown lentils	¼ cup brown lentils
450 ml (16 fl oz) chicken stock	2⅛ cups chicken stock
1 tsp cornflour	1 tsp cornflour

Put the potatoes into an oven preheated to 200°C/400°F/Gas Mark 6 and bake until tender. Heat the oil in a frying pan and fry the pork briskly until well browned. Transfer the meat to a large saucepan. Put the onion, carrots, courgette and mushrooms into the frying pan and fry for a few minutes, then add to the pan with the pork. Season with salt and pepper and add the lentils.

Pour the chicken stock into the frying pan and bring to the boil. Pour the stock over the casserole, bring to the boil, then reduce the heat, cover and simmer for about 40 minutes until the meat is tender.

Mix the cornflour with a little cold water. Stir this mixture into the casserole and cook until thickened. Serve with the baked potatoes.

Low-fat Recipes for Resting the Gallbladder

These recipes are for people wishing to lower the fat content of their diets to help reduce the stimulation of the gall bladder. They are also useful for anyone wishing to lose weight. Use the basic principles and cooking techniques to adapt your own favourite dishes.

Breakfasts

Winter Fruits with Yogurt

3 ready-to-eat apricots	3 ready-to-eat apricots
3 ready-to-eat prunes	3 ready-to-eat prunes
3 ready-to-eat apple slices	3 ready-to-eat apple slices
55 ml (2 fl oz) fresh orange juice	¼ cup fresh orange juice
small pot low-fat plain yogurt	small pot low-fat plain yogurt
2 tbsp crunchy muesli	2 tbsp granola
100 ml (3½ fl oz) skimmed milk	scant ½ cup skim milk

Soak the fruits in the orange juice, plus a little extra water to cover if necessary, overnight.

In the morning, spoon the yogurt over the top and sprinkle on the crunchy muesli. Serve with the skimmed milk.

Pineapple Smoothie and Wholegrain Toast

100 g (4 oz) fresh or tinned pineapple	½ cup fresh or canned pineapple
1 large banana	1 large banana
small pot plain low-fat yogurt	small pot plain low-fat yogurt
2 tbsp crushed ice	2 tbsp crushed ice
1 slice wholemeal bread	1 slice wholewheat bread
1 tsp low-fat spread	1 tsp low-fat spread

Blend together the pineapple, banana and yogurt, then add the crushed ice.

Toast the bread and spread with the low-fat spread.

Grapefruit and Orange Bowl

½ a grapefruit, divided into segments	½ a grapefruit, divided into segments
1 orange, divided into segments	1 orange, divided into segments
2 slices Granary bread	2 slices graham bread
1 tsp low-fat spread	1 tsp low-fat spread
2 tsp jam of your choice	2 tsp jelly of your choice

Mix the grapefruit and orange segments together in a bowl and chill before serving.

Meanwhile, toast the bread and top with the low-fat spread and jam. Serve with the chilled grapefruit and orange.

Toasted Bagel with Cream Cheese and Peaches

1 bagel	1 bagel
1 tbsp cream cheese	1 tbsp cream cheese
1 peach, sliced	1 peach, sliced
200 ml (⅓ pint) orange juice	scant cup orange juice

Slice the bagel in half and toast. Spread with the cream cheese and top with the slices of peach. Serve with a glass of orange juice.

Weetabix, Banana and Toasted Sesame Seeds

2 Weetabix	2 Weetabix
1 large banana, chopped	1 large banana, chopped
½ tsp sesame seeds, toasted	½ tsp sesame seeds, toasted
200 ml (⅓ pint) skimmed milk	scant cup skim milk

Serve the Weetabix with the chopped banana on top. Sprinkle with the sesame seeds and pour the milk over the top.

Lunches

Baked Potatoes with Cottage Cheese

180 g (6 oz) baking potato	6 oz baking potato
110 g (4 oz) cottage cheese	½ cup cottage cheese
handful fresh chives, chopped	handful fresh chives, chopped
1 tomato, chopped	1 tomato, chopped

Pre-heat the oven to 190°C/375°F/gas 5.

Wash the potato, prick it with a fork and bake in the pre-heated oven for 50 minutes, or until it is cooked.

Savoury Scone

90 g (3½ oz) white cabbage, shredded	scant cup shredded white cabbage
1 carrot, grated	1 carrot, shredded
1 apple, grated	1 apple, shredded
2 tbsp reduced-fat salad cream or mayonnaise	2 tbsp reduced-fat salad cream or mayonnaise
1 tbsp raisins	1 tbsp raisins
1 savoury scone	1 savoury biscuit
1 pear	1 pear

Make up some coleslaw by mixing the cabbage with the carrot, apple and salad cream or mayonnaise. Mix in the raisins. Serve the coleslaw with the savoury scone and have the pear for dessert.

Salmon with Beans and Raspberries

60 g (2½ oz) tinned salmon, drained	generous ⅓ cup drained canned salmon
60 g (2½ oz) tinned cannellini beans, drained	½ cup canned drained cannellini beans
50 g (2 oz) tinned broad beans, drained	⅓ cup drained canned fava beans
2 tsp oil-free French dressing	2 tsp oil-free French dressing
1 tbsp chopped fresh flat-leaf parsley	1 tbsp chopped fresh flat-leaf parsley
120 g (4½ oz) chunk French bread	4½ oz chunk French bread
60 g (2½ oz) raspberries or other fresh fruit	½ cup raspberries or other fresh fruit

Mix together the fish and beans. Pour over the dressing and sprinkle the parsley over the top. Serve with the French bread.

Serve the fruit for dessert.

Ham Ploughman's

1 tsp low-fat spread	1 tsp low-fat spread
2 thick slices wholemeal bread	2 thick slices wholewheat bread
80 g (3 oz) ham	3 oz ham
2 large pickled onions	2 large pickled onions
1 apple	1 apple
1 tbsp sweet pickle	1 tbsp relish
1–2 lettuce leaves, washed	1–2 lettuce leaves, washed
200 ml (⅓ pint) tomato juice	scant cup tomato juice
dash of Worcestershire sauce	dash of Worcestershire sauce
1–2 drops Tabasco sauce	1–2 drops hot pepper sauce

Spread the low-fat spread on the bread and then arrange all but the last three ingredients on a plate. To the tomato juice add each of the sauces to taste and serve with the ploughmans.

Mini Pitta with Hummus and Fruit Salad

1 mini pitta bread	1 mini pitta bread
55 g (2 oz) hummus	4 tbsp hummus
1 small apple	1 small apple
1 small pear	1 small pear
1 small banana	1 small banana
60 g (2½ oz) plain low-fat fromage frais	¼ cup plain low-fat fromage blanc

Warm the pitta and cut it into strips. Serve with the hummus as a dip.

Chop up the apple, pear and banana and mix together with the fromage frais for dessert.

Dinners

Tandoori Chicken with Lemon and Orange Sorbet

SERVES 4

4 x 120 g (4½ oz) chicken breasts	4 x 4½ oz chicken breasts
300 g (11 oz) plain low-fat yogurt	300 g (11 oz) plain low-fat yogurt
1 tbsp olive oil	1 tbsp olive oil
1 tsp ground ginger	1 tsp ground ginger
1 tsp chilli powder	1 tsp chili powder
1 tsp paprika	1 tsp paprika

2 cloves garlic, crushed	2 cloves garlic, crushed
2 tbsp tomato purée	2 tbsp tomato paste
240 g (9 oz) brown rice	1¼ cups brown rice
lemon slices and a few sprigs of chopped, fresh parsley, to garnish	lemon slices and a few sprigs of fresh parsley, chopped, to garnish
400 g (14 oz) lemon sorbet	14 oz lemon sorbet
2 oranges, peeled and cut into segments	2 oranges, peeled and cut into segments

Remove the skin from the chicken breasts. Mix together the yogurt, olive oil, ginger, chilli powder, paprika, garlic and tomato purée. Coat the chicken with the mixture and leave, covered, in the fridge to marinate for 10 hours.

When ready to cook, grill each side for 15 minutes.

Meanwhile, cook the brown rice, drain and stir in some of the parsley. Garnish with the lemon and remaining parsley.

For dessert, have the sorbet topped with the orange segments.

Ruby Grapefruit and Tarragon Sole with Baked Apple and Custard

SERVES 4

4 x 100 g (4 oz) lemon sole fillets, skinned	4 x 4 oz sole fillets, skinned
zest of ½ a grapefruit	zest of ½ a grapefruit
½ grapefruit	½ grapefruit
150 g (5 oz) cottage cheese	generous ½ cup cottage cheese
4 spring onions, roughly chopped	4 scallions, roughly chopped
2 tsp chopped fresh tarragon	2 tsp chopped fresh tarragon
salt and freshly ground black pepper	salt and freshly ground black pepper

750 g (1½ lb) potatoes, peeled	1½ lb potatoes, peeled
2 tbsp cornflour	2 tbsp cornstarch
200 g (7 oz) mangetout	7 oz snowpeas
4 large baking apples	4 large tart apples
40 g (1½ oz) demerara sugar	¼ cup coarse light brown sugar
20 g (¾ oz) raisins	1 tbsp raisins
30 g (1 oz) almonds, toasted	¼ cup almonds, toasted
pinch of mixed spice	pinch of pie spice
600 ml (1 pint) ready-to-serve low-fat custard	2½ cups ready-to-serve low-fat custard

Place the fillets in a pan with the grapefruit zest. Cover with water and simmer for about 7 minutes until tender.

While the fish is cooking, cut the grapefruit segments from the pith. Place the cottage cheese, spring onions, tarragon, salt and pepper in a blender and blend until smooth.

When it is ready, transfer the fish, reserving the cooking juices, to a heatproof dish and keep warm.

Boil the potatoes until tender. Blend 175 ml (6 fl oz/¾ cup) of the reserved juices with the cornflour. Stir in a pan over a medium heat until the mixture thickens into a sauce. Also, cook the mangetout. Arrange a fillet of sole on each of four serving plates and pour the sauce over. Serve the potatoes and mangetout.

To make the dessert, pre-heat the oven to 180°C/350°F/gas 4. Core the baking apples, cut a quarter of the core off the bottom of each one and use these as stoppers in the bottoms of the apples to stop the filling running out. Run a sharp knife round the middle of all the skins. Fill the centres with a mix of the sugar, raisins, almonds and mixed spice. Place in a baking dish with 3 table-spoons of water and and bake in the pre-heated oven for 45 minutes to 1 hour, until they are soft all the way through. Heat up the custard and serve with the apples.

Lamb with Raspberry Sauce and Rice Pudding

SERVES 4

4 x 90 g (3½ oz) extra lean lamb fillets	4 x 3½ oz extra lean lamb fillets
600 g (1¼ lb) potatoes	1¼ lb potatoes
knob of margarine or butter	pat of margarine or butter
100 ml (3½ fl oz) skimmed milk	½ cup skim milk
salt and freshly ground black pepper	salt and freshly ground black pepper
300 g (11 oz) tinned raspberries in syrup	2¼ cups canned raspberries in syrup
large sprig of rosemary	large sprig of rosemary
1 tsp dried rosemary, ground	1 tsp dried rosemary, ground
2 tsp cornflour	2 tsp cornstarch
600 g (1¼ lb) tinned low-fat rice pudding or home-made with skimmed milk	1¼ lb canned low-fat rice pudding or home-made with skim milk
12 tinned prunes	12 canned prunes

Grill the lamb fillets for 8 minutes on each side. Peel, chop and boil the potatoes, drain and mash with the margarine or butter and milk and season well.

Heat the raspberries with their syrup together with the rosemary and ground rosemary. Mix the cornflour with a little water in a cup and add to the raspberries. Stir over a medium heat until the syrup has thickened and pour over the grilled lamb. Serve with the mashed potatoes.

For dessert, heat the rice pudding and serve with 3 prunes each.

Oven-baked Mackerel-stuffed Mushrooms and Banana Split

SERVES 4

4 large flat mushrooms	4 large flat mushrooms
185 g (6½ oz) tinned mackerel in mustard sauce	6½ oz canned mackerel in mustard sauce
½ tsp curry powder	½ tsp curry powder
salt and freshly ground black pepper	salt and freshly ground black pepper
2 spring onions, chopped	2 scallions, chopped
2 tbsp chopped fresh parsley	2 tbsp chopped fresh parsley
4 x 120 g (4½ oz) chunks French stick	4 x 4½ oz chunks French stick
4 bananas	4 bananas
240 g (9 oz) reduced-calorie raspberry ripple ice-cream	9 oz reduced-calorie raspberry ripple ice-cream

Pre-heat the oven to 180°C/350°F/gas 4.

Wipe the mushrooms, cut off the stalks and chop them. Place the mushroom caps dark side up on a large piece of foil. Mix the mackerel with the mushroom stalks and curry powder and season to taste. Add the spring onions and half the fresh parsley. Pile the mixture into the mushroom caps. If there is any left, just pile it on the foil to the side. Pull the foil up to encase the stuffed mushrooms and bake in the pre-heated oven for 30 minutes.

Heat the bread. Sprinkle the remaining parsley over the mushrooms before serving with the bread.

For dessert, serve each person with a banana, split lengthways, with 60 g (2½ oz) each of ice-cream spread between the two halves.

Stir-fried Chilli Pork

SERVES 4

450 g (1 lb) extra lean pork	1 lb extra lean pork
10 g (¼ oz) muscovado sugar	1 tbsp dark brown sugar
1 clove of garlic, crushed	1 clove of garlic, minced
pinch of five spice powder	pinch of five spice powder
½ tsp ground cumin	½ tsp ground cumin
240 g (9 oz) brown rice	1¼ cups brown rice
175 g (6 oz) broccoli	6 oz calabrese
2 tbsp olive oil	2 tbsp olive oil
1 yellow pepper, seeded and chopped	1 yellow bell pepper, seeded and chopped
100 g (4 oz) mushrooms, wiped and chopped	2 cups wiped and chopped mushrooms
1 onion, sliced	1 onion, sliced
1 tbsp water	1 tbsp water
100 g (4 oz) tinned water chestnuts, drained	4 oz canned water chestnuts,
dash of soy sauce	dash of soy sauce
handful chives, chopped	handful chives, chopped

Cut the pork into thin slices. Mix the muscovado sugar with the garlic, a good pinch of five spice powder and the cumin. Put the sugar mixture in a dish with the pork and mix well. Leave for 30 minutes.

Meanwhile, cook the brown rice according to the instructions on the pack. While it is cooking, prepare the broccoli by breaking it into small florets and blanch them for 1 minute in boiling water.

Index